Activities to Do with Your Parent Who Has Alzheimer's Dementia

JUDITH A. LEVY, EdM, OTR

CONTENTS

MEDICAL CONCERNS, WHAT YOU SHOULD DO FIRST...

*A*lzheimer's disease is just one of many types of dementias. Any number of underlying medical conditions, diet deficiencies, or even hereditary influences may cause decreasing memory, cognitive problems, or both. Your parent (or even you) might have ignored, or even denied, that any changes have occurred. You need to find out.

When you first notice differences in your parent's behavior and functional skills, the first step you should take is to schedule a visit with his or her physician. Here are some suggestions to help you be prepared for this appointment:

- Write down your questions beforehand. If you think you will remember to ask them all, you are better than I am. Doctors are often pressured for time, your parent might be nervous, you might be stressed, and you might not remember to ask everything you wanted until after you have left the office.

- If the doctor gives permission bring a tape recorder with you to the visit. This step allows you to replay the answers at a later time. When your other family members question you about what the doctor said, this allows you to give reliable responses. If you don't have a recorder, take written notes.

- If you don't understand what the doctor is telling you, ask him or her to explain. That is the reason you are there. Make sure you understand all the words being used.

- If your doctor requires your parent to have further testing, arrange for an in-office, follow-up appointment. At that time you can discuss the results and any future medical plans that may be required. Having this conversation over the phone may seem more convenient, but if possible, a face-to-face visit affords an easier venue for questioning. And again, consider recording this session.

PREFACE

My mother will be ninety-seven years old this coming August. She was diagnosed with dementia when she was eighty-eight. In hindsight her symptoms—missing appointments, getting lost when driving, forgetting birthdays—appeared much sooner, but we failed to make the connection. No one in her personal family history had experienced "senile dementia," as it was previously called, and none of her other relatives had lived past their eighties. So it wasn't something we even considered. We have now been dealing with her decline for nine years, and I don't know how much longer she will live. While she is still my mother she is no longer capable of acting as my mom.

Personally, I have worked as an occupational therapist for more than forty years. I have worked in geriatric care centers and performed home care. I have established programs in hospitals. I have taught home-health aides in a school. I have worked with children and adults suffering from strokes, fractures, as well as arm and hand injuries. In each instance I was the clinician, not the child of the patient. The major difference now is this: this patient doesn't leave at the end of the session, and I cannot go home at the end of the day and leave it all behind. Now *I* am the child, and this is *my* parent. I'm no longer the professional. I have no choice but to adjust to the changes that are happening to her and how they are affecting me. This situation is most difficult since I am no longer objective.

My mother and my family are fortunate that she can afford a full-time caretaker. Her aide is a nice woman who is concerned with helping her maintain the skills she has left. She is receptive to any ideas I might offer. With the use of activities, I feel I'm providing the necessary stimulation my mother needs to continue thinking and "being." My therapy background has become useful in the following way: I can use it to show the caretaker activities that will help challenge my mother, enabling her to spend what time she has left in a purposeful way. I want and need her to function not to just sit and await her demise.

I think of dementia as the "onion disease." Layer by layer it has been peeling off the essence of my mother. It has taken her skills, her independence, and her memory (which now lasts less than twenty seconds). Though she no longer has the senses of smell or taste, she has a great appetite. Though recent cataract surgery has helped her vision and depth perception, she is no longer able to read or comprehend. Her endurance is now poor, and frequent rest stops are required while walking, yet she still wants to go to the mall. Her hearing on the right side is nonexistent, but she is quite capable of hearing from the left side. She is still able to discern sarcasm. Her sense of humor remains intact. She is happy. She told her aide that "as long as she has her health, she is just fine."

The following questions must now be answered: How do I, as the child or caretaker, find an activity that will be challenging without being demeaning? How can I spend my time with her in the most meaningful way?

ACTIVITY SETUP

Being consistent about where and when you do an activity with your parent is important. People with dementia are mentally sharper in the morning. They are more responsive and capable of performing and succeeding with tasks at that time. As the day goes on and draws nearer to dusk, "sundowning" occurs. This frequently seen symptom of dementia is evidenced by an increase in confusion and agitation as daylight diminishes.

I have found it best for my mother to work through several fifteen-minute activities right after breakfast for a total of approximately one hour. After that, I move on to other more physically active skills. The activities I have described in this book are meant to be enjoyable. Should they cause your parent frustration, stop and move on to another one.

We do tasks at the same place each time. Choose a well-lit table with enough space to spread out any items. Make sure the chair where your parent is sitting is comfortable. Ensure that his or her feet reach the floor. If sitting balance is inadequate and your parent tends to lean to one side, be sure to use a chair with arms. If your parent uses a wheelchair, you may pull it up to the table. If it doesn't fit under the table, use a lapboard as the work surface.

Clear the tabletop of other objects so there are few distractions. Turning off the television or radio further decreases the impulse to look around and helps your parent maintain focus on the task you are asking him or her to do. Preferably the tabletop should be opaque, not clear glass. This measure will ensure that the items you are working with are not "lost" in the background of knees or patterned floor coverings. Because my mother has a glass-topped table, we have compensated by placing a towel over the surface. This step helps prevent objects from rolling off the table to the floor, and it offers another cue to her that we are about to do an activity. I use a dark towel when working with light-colored objects and a white towel when working with dark objects. The color contrast allows her to more easily see what she is doing.

Something to consider when setting up activities is where you should be seated. If your parent has decreased peripheral vision, place yourself directly across the table from him or her. This position will keep you within his or her visual field. It will also allow your parent to see you at all times as he or she completes the tasks.

An issue that affects my mother is her inability to hear out of her right ear. Counter intuitively, I place myself on her right side, encouraging her to turn her head to the right to see and hear me. This measure also reinforces her looking toward that side, which she might otherwise ignore. I repeatedly touch her right arm and tap the table, again cuing her to check the right side.

Another area to be concerned about is how you speak with your parent while he or she is doing an activity. Remember, in most cases your parent is trying to please you. He or she might struggle to do what you ask as comprehension becomes more and more difficult. In your parent's past, everything might have come easily to him or her; with the onset of dementia, however, you will find that this ease has markedly changed. He or she will become frustrated, as will you. Your parent will try hard to succeed at what you ask him or her to do, so step back and take a deep breath. Offer directions in simple one- to two-step commands, repeating them as needed to help stimulate his or her memory. Don't forget to offer words of praise. Tell him or her, "What a good job you have done" or "I am proud of you." This reinforcement will go a long way toward his or her success.

If your parent remains frustrated with an activity you have chosen to do, stop. Assess what you are doing. Why isn't it working? Is your parent hungry or physically uncomfortable? Is it a beautiful day? Would he or she rather be outside? Is he or she too tired? Does your parent just not like what you are offering? Ask him or her. Though your parent may have dementia, he or she still has opinions.

Some activities I have included might seem juvenile to you; however, I have found that my mother enjoys doing them. Try them. What's important is that the activities are familiar and stimulate long-term memory. Lastly, I created most of the tasks included within these pages with my mother in mind; however, they are meant to be gender neutral, suitable for both males and females.

I offer an assessment sheet after each activity. It can be used to help document how well the activity went. Also, it can remind you of whether something didn't work well and how you changed it. Use it as a framework for teaching someone else what to do, enabling consistency when he or she acts as your replacement.

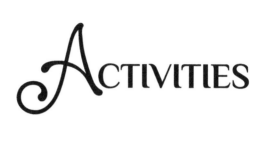

ACTIVITIES

THE ALPHABET

This is a simple place to start. Begin with the letter A and say the letters of the alphabet sequentially all the way to Z. You might think this is something you shouldn't do with your parent—you may think it's too juvenile or that he or she will resent you for offering it. But think again; it isn't. It's familiar, it's rote, and the singsong tempo that comes when you sing it is something your parent might find easy to do. The alphabet is part of his or her long-term memory and can be satisfying if you sing along. High-five your parent when he or she has successfully completed it.

I started my quest looking for magnetic letters of the alphabet. This is the type children use that can be put on the refrigerator, but I couldn't locate them at my local toy store. I did find brightly colored gel alphabet letters at a store called Amazing Savings. My daughter warned me against using them, saying that the gel material would become sticky and attract dirt. But I like them. The colors (red, orange, green, blue, and yellow) were vibrant, and the cost was reasonable. Why not try?

What was an unexpected surprise, however, was that the letters came packaged between two clear plastic sheets. I figured this would keep the letters clean, so I decided to leave them that way. What I did was cut them into squares so each letter remained encased in plastic and could still be manipulated individually. The system worked well. I purchased a large sheet of white paper to put on the tabletop to provide contrast. As a result of keeping the plastic over the letters, I was able to easily move them across the surface.

We sorted the letters by color and then counted which group contained the greatest number. Then we arranged them alphabetically, a task that required verbal cueing from me. Suggestions I offered my mother included, "The *A* is yellow. Can you find it?" When she became stumped, trying to come up with the next letter in the sequence, we returned to singing "The Alphabet Song," and I stopped before the letter she was struggling to remember. This plan worked. Finally, when I asked her to tell me a word for each letter of the alphabet, some of her words were surprising. For example, for the letter *E*, I expected her to say "egg," but she offered "experience."

When we completed these tasks, my mother put the letters alphabetically back into the container. She was thrilled with her success.

Assess This Activity

Date: _____

Name of activity:

_____

Setup location (inside, outside, at a table, in which room):

_____

Setup requirements (where you sat, where your parent sat, type of chairs used, table covering, lighting, any necessary equipment used):

_____

_____

_____

Time of day the activity was done (morning, afternoon, before or after a meal):

_____

Length of time spent at the activity:

_____

Was the activity successful? Did your parent like doing it? Did you?

_____

_____

Did you have to tweak the activity to make it work better for you or your parent? If so, describe how:

_____

_____

Did you teach another person how to do this activity, ensuring you weren't the only one to do it? If so, who?

_____

Would you do this activity again? Yes or no? Why or why not

_____

_____

_____

BAKING

The aroma of something baking in the oven is incomparable. The sense of smell can trigger memories of events from years ago and offer a source of comfort. Baking can often be a way to get your parent talking about his or her favorite foods, childhood holidays, and an event in the past when he or she might have eaten something delicious. I know it has stimulated talks about my grandmother's fantastic apple and cherry pies—particularly that she never measured anything; she innately knew how much of each ingredient to add.

The act of baking itself is structured. It is sequential, time limited, and just plain satisfying. Plus it is always good to have something tasty to eat when you're finished.

If your parent is capable, after washing his or her hands in preparation, have him or her look in the kitchen and help locate needed utensils and additional items. If your parent is unable, let him or her become involved when it comes time to mix the ingredients. Stirring the batter is a good task to get him or her actively moving their arms. Once the item goes into the oven, set the timer. Use the baking time to review what you were doing.

When the timer signals, again reinforce what you have just completed.

If you have made cupcakes, icing them is fun. Different sprinkles can be added too—any design is appreciated. There is no wrong way to decorate a cupcake.

Today, there are many boxed mixes on supermarket shelves that require only a few additional ingredients. Corn muffins, brownies, cupcakes, and cakes are just a few of the myriad choices. Prepared icing really is the icing on the cake. Your parent can bake a treat, ice it, and then have the children or grandchildren over to celebrate.

This is an activity that guarantees success.

Assess This Activity

Date: _____

Name of activity:

_____

Setup location (inside, outside, at a table, in which room):

_____

Setup requirements (where you sat, where your parent sat, type of chairs used, table covering, lighting, any necessary equipment used):

_____

_____

_____

Time of day the activity was done (morning, afternoon, before or after a meal):

_____

Length of time spent at the activity:

_____

Was the activity successful? Did your parent like doing it? Did you?

_____

_____

Did you have to tweak the activity to make it work better for you or your parent? If so, describe how:

_____

_____

Did you teach another person how to do this activity, ensuring you weren't the only one to do it? If so, who?

_____

Would you do this activity again? Yes or no? Why or why not

_____

_____

_____

BALL TOSS

I have seen bean bag toss games and thought this would be a great activity for my mother. With tweaking it can be easily applied to any parent's skill level. I have changed the tossed item from a bean bag, which is floppy and sometimes difficult to control, to a twelve-inch ball. This is bulkier and requires use of both arms and hands. We toss the ball into a laundry basket, and when I want to make it more challenging, we toss it into a large soup pot or a (clean) garbage pail.

Before playing, it is necessary to determine your parent's standing balance. To be safe and appropriate, you must first consider his or her individual needs. If your parent has stable balance, play this activity from a standing position. You can keep a chair nearby if needed. If he or she tends to fall to the side, consider playing from a chair with arms. If he or she uses a walker, use a smaller ball that can be held in one hand. Have him or her hold onto the center crossbar of the walker with one hand for stability and toss the ball with the other hand. If your parent uses a wheelchair, that's fine too. He or she can play from a seated position. Be aware of your parent's endurance level. Should he or she fatigue, remind him or her to take a breather.

My mother and I keep score. I write with a dark marker on bright, white paper and list each point. I encourage my mother to do the addition as we go. When she gets tired or decides she has had enough, we stop. She then totals the numbers to determine the winner. We high-five each other for a game well played.

Assess This Activity

Date: _____

Name of activity:

_____

Setup location (inside, outside, at a table, in which room):

_____

Setup requirements (where you sat, where your parent sat, type of chairs used, table covering, lighting, any necessary equipment used):

_____

_____

_____

Time of day the activity was done (morning, afternoon, before or after a meal):

_____

Length of time spent at the activity:

_____

Was the activity successful? Did your parent like doing it? Did you?

_____

_____

Did you have to tweak the activity to make it work better for you or your parent? If so, describe how:

_____

_____

Did you teach another person how to do this activity, ensuring you weren't the only one to do it? If so, who?

_____

Would you do this activity again? Yes or no? Why or why not

_____

_____

_____

THE BEAUTY PARLOR

When my mother was younger, she went to the beauty parlor weekly to have her hair and nails done. The routine was part of who she was. She enjoyed the personal attention and pampering. They were part of her self-care routine, which made her feel good about herself and how she presented herself to the community at large. We continue to offer this to her now.

Many years have passed, but my mother still goes to the same salon. The same hairdresser and manicurist continue to take care of her. The woman who works at the registration desk is the same as well. I have made it a point to know all these people. They are my security checks on how things are progressing, both with my mother's care and/or behavior as well as with the aide's performance. If they notice any changes, they give me a call.

All this time the women who have had their scheduled appointments, both before and after her, have been consistent. This consistency provides another routine for her and again another security check for me. She no longer can recall their names, yet she knows they look familiar and therefore says hello. Because she is comfortable and feels safe in this routine, I'm comfortable as well.

I have already made arrangements for when my mother is unable to go to the beauty parlor. The hairdresser has told me she will attend to her at home.

Assess This Activity

Date: _____

Name of activity:

_____

Setup location (inside, outside, at a table, in which room):

_____

Setup requirements (where you sat, where your parent sat, type of chairs used, table covering, lighting, any necessary equipment used):

_____

_____

_____

Time of day the activity was done (morning, afternoon, before or after a meal):

_____

Length of time spent at the activity:

_____

Was the activity successful? Did your parent like doing it? Did you?

_____

_____

Did you have to tweak the activity to make it work better for you or your parent? If so, describe how:

_____

_____

Did you teach another person how to do this activity, ensuring you weren't the only one to do it? If so, who?

_____

Would you do this activity again? Yes or no? Why or why not

_____

_____

_____

BINGO

It seems like the game of Bingo is everywhere—from schools to churches and Indian casinos. It appeals to all ages and across all cultures. It is social.

Bingo can be adapted for individuals struggling with limited vision by enlarging the size of the print on the cards. It may also be adapted for those with fine hand coordination problems by using a thick marker pen to mark spots. Marking is also easier than using cards which require you to slide a plastic disk over each square. The disk may move and cause confusion.

Bingo may be played from a seated or standing position. No game lasts overly long, and you may stop without affecting another player should your parent's attention span start to wander.

If you further evaluate the game of Bingo, you will realize it is also a great game for those struggling with mild-to-moderate dementia. It enhances concentration and listening skills. As the leader calls out each letter or number combination, your parent must search his or her own specific Bingo card to establish whether it is there. This exercise stimulates memory since your parent must remember that just-called combination from the time it was announced to the time he or she locates it on the card. Your parent must retain that information as he or she marks the designated spot before moving on to the next-called combination.

Bingo worked for my mother until it didn't. I knew I had to change how we used the Bingo set when her frustration level grew too quickly, she was no longer interested, and it no longer provided a positive experience. At this time we use the game for matching. We place all the balls into a bowl. As we select each one, my mother has to locate its space on the master sheet and then correctly place the ball in it. We continue until she gets tired, and then we move on to another task.

Assess This Activity

Date: _____

Name of activity:

_____

Setup location (inside, outside, at a table, in which room):

_____

Setup requirements (where you sat, where your parent sat, type of chairs used, table covering, lighting, any necessary equipment used):

_____

_____

_____

Time of day the activity was done (morning, afternoon, before or after a meal):

_____

Length of time spent at the activity:

_____

Was the activity successful? Did your parent like doing it? Did you?

_____

_____

Did you have to tweak the activity to make it work better for you or your parent? If so, describe how:

_____

_____

Did you teach another person how to do this activity, ensuring you weren't the only one to do it? If so, who?

_____

Would you do this activity again? Yes or no? Why or why not

_____

_____

_____

BLOWING BUBBLES

This is a pleasant way to spend some time. Blowing bubbles is easy to do and often brings back childhood memories. What can be better than following the path of a bubble before it bursts? You can sit outside on your patio or even take a lawn chair and go out to your backyard. Remember, if you are going outside, have your parent dress appropriately. The elderly are often more susceptible to cold than those who are younger.

This activity is repetitive and fun and good for the following: eye-hand coordination, breath control, increasing lung capacity, and visual tracking. It can be done from a seated or standing position. If one is standing, it encourages endurance, standing tolerance, and good balance. Have your parent stand as long as he or she can but place a chair nearby for when he or she wants to sit down.

Before beginning, consider pouring the bubble liquid into a wide-mouthed container or pan so it affords easy access for the bubble wand. I have also filled a large pot with water and had my mother blow the bubbles into the water. They will remain there longer. She can pop them too, bringing in the skill of eye-hand coordination.

If your parent can blow the bubbles, let him or her. Just remember—if this activity causes your parent to become short of breath, it's time to stop and alter how you have set up the task. Instead of "blowing" the bubbles, have your parent wave the bubble wand across his or her body creating the wind, which will make the bubbles. Or, if your parent becomes tired, you can take control over the bubble wand. If you blow more slowly, you will create a larger bubble, one that can be more visible and easier for your parent to track. You may also consider an automated bubble gun. These toys make large clusters of bubbles, which are more visible.

Today's bubble innovators have even created a special liquid that makes colored bubbles. Your parent may see them more easily, and you can consider trying them.

Playing with bubbles is a good activity to do with grand-children. Sometimes when they come to visit, you can be stumped when planning your time. This one encourages interaction in a positive way.

Assess This Activity

Date: _____

Name of activity:

_____

Setup location (inside, outside, at a table, in which room):

_____

Setup requirements (where you sat, where your parent sat, type of chairs used, table covering, lighting, any necessary equipment used):

_____

_____

_____

Time of day the activity was done (morning, afternoon, before or after a meal):

_____

Length of time spent at the activity:

_____

Was the activity successful? Did your parent like doing it? Did you?

_____

_____

Did you have to tweak the activity to make it work better for you or your parent? If so, describe how:

_____

_____

Did you teach another person how to do this activity, ensuring you weren't the only one to do it? If so, who?

_____

Would you do this activity again? Yes or no? Why or why not

_____

_____

_____

BUTTONS

Everyone has them lying around the corners of his or her drawers. Buttons are just waiting to be put to use. And since they come in a multitude of colors and sizes, they are perfect for sorting. I have found that the best buttons are large and made of one color.

Before you begin, place a towel on the surface of your worktable. This will help prevent the buttons from falling onto the floor. Separate them by colors or sort them by size. You can count which color has the greatest or fewest amount. You can fill containers by color and then pour them out. You can form the buttons into rows or even make them into circles to create smiley faces. My mother and I have also placed them into descending-size order.

If your parent wants to copy your designs, make yours to his or her left and have your parent copy his or hers to the right side. Designs may be made from straight lines, intersecting lines, triangles, squares, or circles. You can form the outline of a shape in one color and then fill it in with a different-colored button. Do not limit yourself to just simple designs—you can make trees, bodies, and faces. Let your imagination go.

Another activity I have done, requires my mother to hold four to five buttons in the palm of her closed hand. Using just that hand she has to manipulate each button to place it, one at a time, into a container without dropping it. Should she drop one, she has to start over. This activity encourages counting, eye-hand coordination, and concentration to do it successfully. A similar task can be achieved by putting a coin into the slot of a piggy bank.

I have spent a lot of time with my mother making letters of the alphabet from buttons. We have also created the letters needed to spell her name. I form the letters to her left, and she copies them to her right. Initially, I thought she might be upset with this activity; surprisingly she was quite pleased as she completed it.

Assess This Activity

Date: _____

Name of activity:

_____

Setup location (inside, outside, at a table, in which room):

_____

Setup requirements (where you sat, where your parent sat, type of chairs used, table covering, lighting, any necessary equipment used):

_____

_____

_____

Time of day the activity was done (morning, afternoon, before or after a meal):

_____

Length of time spent at the activity:

_____

Was the activity successful? Did your parent like doing it? Did you?

_____

_____

Did you have to tweak the activity to make it work better for you or your parent? If so, describe how:

_____

_____

Did you teach another person how to do this activity, ensuring you weren't the only one to do it? If so, who?

_____

Would you do this activity again? Yes or no? Why or why not

_____

_____

_____

CATEGORIES

Categories is a game you might have played with your friends or siblings when you were younger. Our family used to play it in the car to pass the time while we were traveling to our destination. Today I play it with my grandchildren.

The object is to choose a general topic and then take turns listing all the items included in it. To remain in the game, you must remember the previously listed items. If you duplicate one that was already stated, you are eliminated. The loser is the one who can no longer think of an item. The winner is the last one to list an item for that category. Some categories might include types of flowers, types of dogs, types of vegetables, names of colors, and names of states. The categories are endless.

Today I play two variations of this game with my mother. Needless to say, she doesn't have to recall any of the previously listed words, and she isn't eliminated should she duplicate a word. We have no winners and no losers.

The first way we play is to write the category on the top of a piece of paper. I continue to write her list of items as she states them. This way she can refer back as necessary. I frequently remind her of the topic and reread aloud her list as a cue. My goal is to find two to three items in each chosen category.

The second way requires a little more planning on my part. I have preselected a category along with three to four items included in it. I have written each word on separate index cards. Included are two words that do not fit the category. My mother is responsible for selecting the correct words, separating out those that don't belong. The television program *Sesame Street* offers a variation on Categories with its song: "Which of these things is not like the other? Which of these things is just not the same?"

Again, like most other activities for your parent, if he or she displays frustration and decides he or she has had enough, stop and move on to another task.

Assess This Activity

Date: _____

Name of activity:

_____

Setup location (inside, outside, at a table, in which room):

_____

Setup requirements (where you sat, where your parent sat, type of chairs used, table covering, lighting, any necessary equipment used):

_____

_____

_____

Time of day the activity was done (morning, afternoon, before or after a meal):

_____

Length of time spent at the activity:

_____

Was the activity successful? Did your parent like doing it? Did you?

_____

_____

Did you have to tweak the activity to make it work better for you or your parent? If so, describe how:

_____

_____

Did you teach another person how to do this activity, ensuring you weren't the only one to do it? If so, who?

_____

Would you do this activity again? Yes or no? Why or why not

_____

_____

_____

Coloring Books

I like children's coloring books. The pictures are of familiar and easily recognized objects. The presented designs are drawn in clear black and white that are easily seen, even if your parent has decreased vision. This activity can stimulate your parent's memory, verbal or word-finding skills, eye-hand coordination, and color discrimination. It can reinforce decision making as well.

To start, be sure you are seated at a table with a bright light. Begin by looking through the book together. Have your parent name and describe the pictures he or she sees. You can then have your parent choose, if he or she is able, the picture he or she would like to color. I like to tear out the selected page and place it on the table. It is easier to color a page that is resting flat on a surface, and this step prevents the book from closing on your parent's hands as he or she draws.

I have located large, triangular crayons, made by Melissa & Doug, which I prefer to use. Their shape prevents them from rolling off the table, their size makes them easier to hold, and their bright, vivid colors make them easy to find. These are perfect for those individuals who suffer decreased vision or arthritic hands. Before we begin, we discuss the names of the colors and which one is the appropriate choice for the picture she has chosen. Initially, my mother was able to choose which crayon she wanted; now, as her dementia has progressed, she requires a cue to make any decisions.

Consequently, I pick the crayon, and she begins to color. She determines when she is done with the picture. Once she is finished, we review what we have done together. She labels the colors she used and describes the picture. I ask her to spell the name of the object in the picture as I write the name alongside the graphic. We then tape her pictures to the wall near where she sits and refer back to them throughout the day.

Assess This Activity

Name of activity:

_____

Setup location (inside, outside, at a table, in which room):

_____

Setup requirements (where you sat, where your parent sat, type of chairs used, table covering, lighting, any necessary equipment used):

_____

_____

_____

Time of day the activity was done (morning, afternoon, before or after a meal):

_____

Length of time spent at the activity:

_____

Was the activity successful? Did your parent like doing it? Did you?

_____

_____

Did you have to tweak the activity to make it work better for you or your parent? If so, describe how:

_____

_____

Did you teach another person how to do this activity, ensuring you weren't the only one to do it? If so, who?

_____

Would you do this activity again? Yes or no? Why or why not

_____

_____

_____

Cooking

y mother was the one in our family who shopped for groceries as well as prepped and made the meals. Included in her recipe collection was chicken soup. She had been eating it since childhood. I decided to make some soup one morning before visiting her, and since I brought some with me and it was a familiar food for her, I thought it might be a good activity for her to list the ingredients that made soup "soup." As the saying goes...it couldn't hurt.

This was one of the more difficult tasks I had asked of her. It required all her memory skills for completion and necessitated many verbal cues from me. I asked her to list ingredients, and she was able to mention bones. That was it. I was able to get more items specified by asking general questions, such as the following: What makes chicken soup "chicken soup"? Are there any vegetables we should use? Can you think of an orange- or green-colored vegetable we might include? What makes it wet? Should we put in seasonings? If so, which ones?

While this was a good activity and one that can be applied to any familiar food your parent has prepared in the past, I made a mistake in how I presented this task to her. It was frustrating for me, and it would have been more successful if I had planned ahead. I should have offered pictures of all items to be included in the recipe as well as pictures of extra items that didn't belong. That way she could have selected the correct ones. Also, my mother would have had an easier time if I had written down the ingredients as she listed them instead of my presenting them all orally.

I still think this is a good activity. It can be applied to any food that is familiar to your parent. Next time I try this, I will consider recipes for foods that require only one to two items (for example, chocolate milk or apple sauce) instead of those with multiple ingredients (such as cakes or omelets or chicken soup).

At this time my mother still shows an interest in cooking but her role has changed to that of observer. She sits in the kitchen and enjoys the aromas of foods as they cook. We discuss each ingredient as we add them to our dishes. This offers another opportunity for conversation. We describe the dinner that she is about to eat and we reminisce about the meals that she created in the past.

Assess This Activity

Date: _____

Name of activity:

_____

Setup location (inside, outside, at a table, in which room):

_____

Setup requirements (where you sat, where your parent sat, type of chairs used, table covering, lighting, any necessary equipment used):

_____

_____

_____

Time of day the activity was done (morning, afternoon, before or after a meal):

_____

Length of time spent at the activity:

_____

Was the activity successful? Did your parent like doing it? Did you?

_____

_____

Did you have to tweak the activity to make it work better for you or your parent? If so, describe how:

_____

_____

Did you teach another person how to do this activity, ensuring you weren't the only one to do it? If so, who?

_____

Would you do this activity again? Yes or no? Why or why not

_____

_____

_____

Counting

My mother and I count everything: coins, buttons, sugar packets, playing cards, even spools of thread. They are all items we can and have counted. With counting there is only one precise answer. If your parent makes a mistake, you can recount until the answer is correct.

Counting objects is a concrete skill. For those who have dementia, mental acuity can vary from day to day. This condition affects the quantity of items I offer for her to count. On bad days we count fewer items, sometimes only up to ten. On exceptionally good days when she appears to have better cognition, we might count to one hundred. She might even count by twos or tens.

I like counting pennies or buttons. We place the uncounted items to the left, and as we count them, we place them in a bowl to the right. This step ensures we haven't counted them twice.

Counting time is an abstract skill that may be too confusing for those with dementia. Your parent may be unable to answer "How many more hours until dinner?" or "How many days until we go to the beauty parlor?"

Restructuring these questions in a more visual way will make them easier to comprehend. For example: "Here's the calendar. Today is Monday. Let's cross off the days until Friday when you will have your hair appointment. We can count how many days that will be."

Some months ago my mother found it easy to count past ten or to count by tens up to one hundred. Now things have changed. While she can still count, she loses track. She requires a cue from me to continue to completion.

Assess This Activity

Date: _____

Name of activity:

_____

Setup location (inside, outside, at a table, in which room):

_____

Setup requirements (where you sat, where your parent sat, type of chairs used, table covering, lighting, any necessary equipment used):

_____

_____

_____

Time of day the activity was done (morning, afternoon, before or after a meal):

_____

Length of time spent at the activity:

_____

Was the activity successful? Did your parent like doing it? Did you?

_____

_____

Did you have to tweak the activity to make it work better for you or your parent? If so, describe how:

_____

_____

Did you teach another person how to do this activity, ensuring you weren't the only one to do it? If so, who?

_____

Would you do this activity again? Yes or no? Why or why not

_____

_____

_____

CROSSWORD PUZZLES

My mother was a brilliant crossword puzzle solver. She started each day with a cup of coffee and her puzzle. She especially looked forward to the Sunday *New York Times* puzzle because it was both clever and challenging. What gratification to complete it! She still enjoys doing crosswords, but now l must alter them to compensate for her decreased vision, her shorter attention span, and her inconsistent comprehension skills.

l have found crossword puzzle books in the supermarket, and we often do them on days when l feel she is especially mentally sharp. We sit at the kitchen table and complete the puzzle together. l read the clue to her and frame it in such a way that she can be successful with the answer. Surprisingly, she is still quite good at this. l then fill in the answer. Sometimes when she is speaking, her word-finding skills are inconsistent, and she gets lost in her sentences. However, when doing crossword puzzles with specific clues offered to her, she somehow figures out the answer and has no difficulty finding the correct word. She might have dementia, but she's still smart!

Often while answering the clue, she segues into another word, and we end up discussing an altogether different topic. She can be really interesting.

Doing a puzzle might be your intention, but it may not be what you end up doing. Be flexible. Put away the crossword puzzle and see where your parent's new direction takes you.

Assess This Activity

Date: _____

Name of activity:

_____

Setup location (inside, outside, at a table, in which room):

_____

Setup requirements (where you sat, where your parent sat, type of chairs used, table covering, lighting, any necessary equipment used):

_____

_____

_____

Time of day the activity was done (morning, afternoon, before or after a meal):

_____

Length of time spent at the activity:

_____

Was the activity successful? Did your parent like doing it? Did you?

_____

_____

Did you have to tweak the activity to make it work better for you or your parent? If so, describe how:

_____

_____

Did you teach another person how to do this activity, ensuring you weren't the only one to do it? If so, who?

_____

Would you do this activity again? Yes or no? Why or why not

_____

_____

_____

Dancing

ancing is a wonderful activity for everyone. It is social and fun. The many benefits include improved circulation, more effective breathing and lung capacity, longer endurance, greater mobility, improved standing tolerance, and increased attention to sequencing skills. I'm sure your first thought was to dance while standing upright; however, this can be adjusted depending on your parent's circumstances. If he or she has poor balance, use a walker. If he or she is confined to a wheelchair, don't despair. Grab your parent's hands and move his or her arms to the rhythm. You might be in for a surprise.

Choose music that was produced during your parent's youth. I didn't think my mother had it in her, but when "Boogie Woogie Bugle Boy of Company B" came on, she was up and ready to dance the lindy! It just took the right incentive.

We have also spent time dancing to "The Hokey Pokey" as well as "Head, Shoulders, Knees, and Toes." My mother is familiar with both songs. At times I have to hold her hands to prevent her from falling, but she's ready to get moving. What I like about "The Hokey Pokey" is that it targets balance, especially when she gets to the part where she has to put her "leg in and shake it all about." Furthermore, the dance helps to reinforce right versus left. What I like about "Head, Shoulders, Knees, and Toes" is that it reinforces body parts. You might feel silly, but your parent will have a good time being with you and get to practice coordination at the same time. You will know it's time to stop dancing when and if he or she—or you—gets short of breath.

There might be a specific dance your parent knows how to do but you do not. Ask him or her to teach you. It's possible that your parent's memory about this dance might come back to him or her.

Dancing with my mother has led to conversations about my father. He was a great dancer known to his friends as Twinkle Toes. In the middle of one 1940's song medley, she began to talk about how she met him. It was at a "Five Star" dance in Newark, New Jersey, in the 1940s. What a nice remembrance it was for her and for me as well.

Assess This Activity

Date: _____

Name of activity:

_____

Setup location (inside, outside, at a table, in which room):

_____

Setup requirements (where you sat, where your parent sat, type of chairs used, table covering, lighting, any necessary equipment used):

_____

_____

_____

Time of day the activity was done (morning, afternoon, before or after a meal):

_____

Length of time spent at the activity:

_____

Was the activity successful? Did your parent like doing it? Did you?

_____

_____

Did you have to tweak the activity to make it work better for you or your parent? If so, describe how:

_____

_____

Did you teach another person how to do this activity, ensuring you weren't the only one to do it? If so, who?

_____

Would you do this activity again? Yes or no? Why or why not

_____

_____

_____

DOLLS

olls bring comfort and offer the ability to nurture. They aren't something I would offer to someone newly diagnosed with dementia but rather for someone in the latter stages of the disease. Seeing your parent interact with a doll as if it were a real baby might make you, the child or caregiver, uncomfortable, but this is usually not the case for your parent. When I was working in geriatric care facilities, dolls were given to the female patients. Today, as more men have taken on the role of child caregivers it is possible they too might benefit from having a doll.

I prefer plain dolls that are large and huggable. Choose those with a natural face as opposed to those with exaggerated features that mimic cartoon characters. The doll's clothing should be easily removed and reapplied without too many buttons or snaps. I also prefer dolls that are washable.

Select those dolls that do not require a battery and that do not "speak" or "cry." It shouldn't be necessary for your parent to respond to the doll's preprogrammed commands.The doll should allow your parent to interact with it as he or she is able.   I also prefer to stay away from stuffed animals because they get dirty and dusty, and are hard to keep clean.

Consider purchasing a doll and leaving it on your parent's bed as a decoration. He or she will choose to hold it or not when he or she is ready. Whether to interact with the doll will be your parent's decision, but you will have provided the opportunity.

Assess This Activity

Date: _____

Name of activity:

_____

Setup location (inside, outside, at a table, in which room):

_____

Setup requirements (where you sat, where your parent sat, type of chairs used, table covering, lighting, any necessary equipment used):

_____

_____

_____

Time of day the activity was done (morning, afternoon, before or after a meal):

_____

Length of time spent at the activity:

_____

Was the activity successful? Did your parent like doing it? Did you?

_____

_____

Did you have to tweak the activity to make it work better for you or your parent? If so, describe how:

_____

_____

Did you teach another person how to do this activity, ensuring you weren't the only one to do it? If so, who?

_____

Would you do this activity again? Yes or no? Why or why not

_____

_____

_____

DOMINOES

Remember these? The wooden black ones with the white spots? They are just perfect! They are the right size to pick up, and the clean black-and-white colors are clearly seen. This is a great find for someone who has vision difficulty. There are so many activities you can do with them.

Put a light-colored cloth or towel on the table surface to provide contrast and pour out the dominoes. Begin by turning them faceup. Collect all the dominoes that have one spot and work your way up to those that have six. See if your parent can find those that have the same number of spots on each side. You can turn the dominoes facedown. What is nice about this game is that it's easy to tell when you're done. Every piece is black. There is a definite conclusion.

Dominoes can be used for building as well. We have constructed two- as well as three-dimensional shapes: squares, rectangles, and teetering pyramids. We have made large circles of dominoes and then formed them into faces. I usually lie the dominoes flat for the circle and turn them on their sides for the hair and nose to add interest. We have a competition to see how tall a tower we each can build before the towers fall over.

Dominoes can be used for forming letters too. Since reading is a left-to-right skill, you should sit at your parent's left side when you form your letter design. Have your parent then make his or her replica to his or her right.

When your parent has had enough, complete the activity by putting the dominoes away. What's convenient is that there's no right or wrong way to replace them in the box. Horizontally or vertically, they fit inside each way just as well. No frustration here—just a good time-limited activity with a defined conclusion.

Assess This Activity

Date: _____

Name of activity:

_____

Setup location (inside, outside, at a table, in which room):

_____

Setup requirements (where you sat, where your parent sat, type of chairs used, table covering, lighting, any necessary equipment used):

_____

_____

_____

Time of day the activity was done (morning, afternoon, before or after a meal):

_____

Length of time spent at the activity:

_____

Was the activity successful? Did your parent like doing it? Did you?

_____

_____

Did you have to tweak the activity to make it work better for you or your parent? If so, describe how:

_____

_____

Did you teach another person how to do this activity, ensuring you weren't the only one to do it? If so, who?

_____

Would you do this activity again? Yes or no? Why or why not

_____

_____

_____

DRAWING

What's so wonderful about drawing is that it's an easy activity to set up. It requires little in the way of supplies and can be done almost anywhere as long as you have a hard surface for support. I like to use bright, white paper since it provides good contrast for any design. The paper can be purchased at any art supply store and is sold in pads with sturdy cardboard backing; it's also good for leaning on. I have amassed a supply of colored pencils, crayons, and markers to provide variety.

Drawing is a decision-making skill for someone with dementia, requiring him or her to choose a color and specific writing implement. This activity might require assistance from you.

Drawing can be done inside at the kitchen table or, weather permitting, outside at a table or even while sitting on a park bench. Your parent is limited to what he or she draws and to how complicated the colors and design will be based on his or her imagination. Look around and choose the subject. If you're outside, it can be a drawing of a tree, flower, or even the grass and sky. If you're inside, you can draw a picture of a clock or chair. If your parent is able to do only simple shapes, then drawing circles or squares is okay as well. Whatever he or she draws is fine. It's the act of drawing, not the finished product, that is important.

My mother has a beanbag jack-o'-lantern toy I gave her one year for Halloween. Bright orange and approximately four inches wide, it has a black triangular hat. She loves it. So that is what we decided to draw. She was unable to initiate the act of drawing, so I went first. Seated to her left, I drew an orange circle. I then gave her the crayon and prompted her to draw an orange circle as well. With a cue, she did just fine. We continued taking turns, progressing to the black crayon for the hat and facial features, until we were finished. With my help she dated and signed her name. Now the picture of this toy hangs on the wall along with other drawings she has done.

Assess This Activity

Name of activity:

_____

Setup location (inside, outside, at a table, in which room):

_____

Setup requirements (where you sat, where your parent sat, type of chairs used, table covering, lighting, any necessary equipment used):

_____

_____

_____

Time of day the activity was done (morning, afternoon, before or after a meal):

_____

Length of time spent at the activity:

_____

Was the activity successful? Did your parent like doing it? Did you?

_____

_____

Did you have to tweak the activity to make it work better for you or your parent? If so, describe how:

_____

_____

Did you teach another person how to do this activity, ensuring you weren't the only one to do it? If so, who?

_____

Would you do this activity again? Yes or no? Why or why not

_____

_____

_____

Folding

Almost anything can be folded. When done while seated at the table, your task can be as simple as folding a piece of paper or laundry. Your parent probably knows how to fold from years of experience, and you may not have to demonstrate folding for him or her. But should he or she not remember and need a cue on how to begin, sit next to your parent and have him or her copy what you do. If your parent tends to ignore his or her right or left side, remember to sit by that affected side. Encourage his or her attention to a complete visual field by tapping his or her ignored side, arm, or tabletop. Once you have his or her interest, you can begin to fold the item into any shape you want: a rectangle, a square, or diagonally into a triangle.

If your parent can stand without support, folding can be done while standing up. A perfect use for this posture is when folding a bed sheet or a large towel. When done this way, folding encourages standing balance as well as endurance. It serves to stretch and strengthen both upper arms. It also helps to improve chest expansion, which is necessary for adequate breathing and helpful for circulation.

I've had my mother fold grocery bags after we've returned from the supermarket. She also enjoys folding the multitude of plastic bags that keep accumulating.

What's nice about this activity is that it's familiar and purposeful. It's repetitive, it takes only a short amount of time, and it has a definite conclusion.

Assess This Activity

Date: _____

Name of activity:

_____

Setup location (inside, outside, at a table, in which room):

_____

Setup requirements (where you sat, where your parent sat, type of chairs used, table covering, lighting, any necessary equipment used):

_____

_____

_____

Time of day the activity was done (morning, afternoon, before or after a meal):

_____

Length of time spent at the activity:

_____

Was the activity successful? Did your parent like doing it? Did you?

_____

_____

Did you have to tweak the activity to make it work better for you or your parent? If so, describe how:

_____

_____

Did you teach another person how to do this activity, ensuring you weren't the only one to do it? If so, who?

_____

Would you do this activity again? Yes or no? Why or why not

_____

_____

_____

GARDENING

When I think about gardening, I think about warmth, summer, and getting down and dirty in the soil to plant vegetables, flowers, or both. I also think about starting with seeds and watching them grow.

These may sound like wonderful activities to do; however, they're not best for someone suffering with dementia. First of all, the weather is often too hot and uncomfortable to be exercising outdoors. Also, for the elderly or even the nonexercising public, squatting or even rising up from ground level isn't easy.

This exercise can be hard on the hip and knee joints, and it might adversely affect blood pressure. Balance when squatting is an iffy proposition too. Finally, waiting for seeds to germinate takes too long, and those with dementia won't be able to remember what they planted, the fact that they planted, or even what they initially wanted to grow. So...what to do?

I've decided to forego vegetables and stick to flats of flowers and herbs. We use raised gardening beds and window planter boxes. Elevating the work area is helpful to prevent unnecessary bending, balance issues, or both. The flowers are lifted from the ground to be at eye level. I also appreciate the limitations of a window planter. This smaller size requires less effort, and the project can be completed in a shorter time—something good to consider if a shortened attention span or fatigue is an issue for your parent.

I prefer to buy almost fully grown flowers from the local nursery or market. I like flowers with large, vivid blooms and select those with good color contrast. This choice makes it easier for them to be seen. A good choice might be red geraniums planted among large-headed yellow marigolds.

When setting up a gardening project, have your parent sit outside at a table with all the needed implements at hand. Have him or her place the flowers into the boxes where he or she wants them. It might be necessary for you to help him or her decide which plant to choose and where the placement should be. You can be responsible for distributing the soil, followed by his or her tamping it down. Your parent can follow up with the watering and pruning of the plants on an ongoing basis as part of his or her after-breakfast routine.

My mother has three planter boxes on her patio railing. Two are filled with flowers. The third has herbs, which we use for cooking as well as for enjoying their aroma. I also like to plant some "cutting" flowers in the window boxes to have for inside arrangements, which we place in vases throughout the apartment. My mother enjoys seeing these flowers around her house. She still manipulates the arrangements to her choosing as she passes by.

Assess This Activity

Date: _____

Name of activity:

_____

Setup location (inside, outside, at a table, in which room):

_____

Setup requirements (where you sat, where your parent sat, type of chairs used, table covering, lighting, any necessary equipment used):

_____

_____

_____

Time of day the activity was done (morning, afternoon, before or after a meal):

_____

Length of time spent at the activity:

_____

Was the activity successful? Did your parent like doing it? Did you?

_____

_____

Did you have to tweak the activity to make it work better for you or your parent? If so, describe how:

_____

_____

Did you teach another person how to do this activity, ensuring you weren't the only one to do it? If so, who?

_____

Would you do this activity again? Yes or no? Why or why not

_____

_____

_____

GETTING DRESSED

The morning routine for someone with dementia often sets the tone for the remainder of the day. Personal hygiene and bathing are a given. They are structured tasks. There are no decisions to make; just take care of business and move on to the next item on the agenda—dressing. That is when your parent's decision-making ability comes into play.

My mother and I first discuss the weather. Will it be cold or hot? Will we stay inside or go out? Do our plans for the day include visitors, or are we just hanging out? The answers to these questions help determine what to wear. We start with underwear and proceed toward outer clothing and accessories. My mother had always been fashion conscious and clothing choices were well thought out, but now she requires assistance in choosing which item she will wear. I still want her to look sharp.

At this time I limit her selection to two choices; then the process is less confusing and stressful. What would she prefer? Black slacks or blue slacks? Which shirt would she favor? White or patterned? I like to offer her options since it continues to involve her in the process. If she's unable to make the choice, I just do it for her; it's unnecessary for her to choose merely to prove she can.

Some individuals who have dementia prefer to wear the same items of clothing everyday. They want to wear them even if soiled; they want what they want when they want it. Do not make a point of explaining why changing clothes is necessary. Just go with it. Purchase multiple sets of the same articles of clothing and while showering your parent, just substitute the clean clothes. Choose your fights wisely! Also, if too many articles of clothing cause contentious behavior, leave out the extras. Wearing that belt or scarf may not be necessary; perhaps it can be applied later in the day.

Assess This Activity

Date: _____

Name of activity:

_____

Setup location (inside, outside, at a table, in which room):

_____

Setup requirements (where you sat, where your parent sat, type of chairs used, table covering, lighting, any necessary equipment used):

_____

_____

_____

Time of day the activity was done (morning, afternoon, before or after a meal):

_____

Length of time spent at the activity:

_____

Was the activity successful? Did your parent like doing it? Did you?

_____

_____

Did you have to tweak the activity to make it work better for you or your parent? If so, describe how:

_____

_____

Did you teach another person how to do this activity, ensuring you weren't the only one to do it? If so, who?

_____

Would you do this activity again? Yes or no? Why or why not

_____

_____

_____

GHOST

Ghost is an interactive game I frequently play with my grandchildren. I have found that my mother is able to participate in playing this game as well.

To play you need a minimum of two participants. Decide who will go first. One way to choose is by rolling dice to see who has the highest or lowest number. If your parent can still count up to twelve, use both dice; if he or she can count only up to six, use a single die. Whoever wins the dice toss will then begin the game by starting with the word *ghost*. The second player must then proffer a word that begins with the last letter of "ghost" (a *T*). His or her choice, for example, might be "tuna fish." The game proceeds as the next player in turn states a word that begins with an *H* (the last letter of "tuna fish"), and so it goes. If you wish, words may be chosen by category, such as animals or colors. Continue playing until you cannot think of another word.

This is a game that stimulates memory. It encourages participants to remember what was just mentioned. It requires focus since they must recall the last letter of the previous word. Only then can the game progress. If your parent is having trouble remembering spoken words, this game may be altered by switching to writing down the words as you go. For the parent with decreased vision, take care to write with a dark pen on bright, white paper so the words are easily seen.

If Ghost proves to be too difficult or your parent no longer shows interest, move on to a different activity.

Assess This Activity

Date: _____

Name of activity:

_____

Setup location (inside, outside, at a table, in which room):

_____

Setup requirements (where you sat, where your parent sat, type of chairs used, table covering, lighting, any necessary equipment used):

_____

_____

_____

Time of day the activity was done (morning, afternoon, before or after a meal):

_____

Length of time spent at the activity:

_____

Was the activity successful? Did your parent like doing it? Did you?

_____

_____

Did you have to tweak the activity to make it work better for you or your parent? If so, describe how:

_____

_____

Did you teach another person how to do this activity, ensuring you weren't the only one to do it? If so, who?

_____

Would you do this activity again? Yes or no? Why or why not

_____

_____

_____

Going Out for a Meal

What a treat for you, the caretaker, and your parent to get out of the house. It's always nice to have a change of scenery and not have to be the one to cook or clean, let alone decide what someone else might want to eat. For someone with dementia, leaving the safe environment of home is always a challenge. Select the right restaurant by ensuring that it's not too noisy or too far, that the lighting is adequate, that the line to be seated won't be too long, and that it won't take overly long for the food to arrive.

Often when we are out, people my mother knew in the past come up to the table to greet her. With some prompting from us, she responds quite well and always says, "Hello. How nice to see you." She's always thrilled to be social.

A few years ago we went to finer restaurants. We thought that would be wonderful. These were locations where my mother would have been thrilled to go in the past. As time went on our emphasis on the "where" had to change, as she did. How quickly we learned that we should have chosen a location for its familiarity, not for its prestige. She no longer required fancy meals but instead needed consistent meals. Also, initially she could order from the menu for herself, but it has now become necessary for us to order meals for her. She eats the same food each time, and each time she is satisfied. We have had the break from our routine we needed.

We often follow dinner at the restaurant with a trip to the ice cream shop for a coffee cone. Each time she says, "I can't remember the last time I had that."

Assess This Activity

Date: _____

Name of activity:

_____

Setup location (inside, outside, at a table, in which room):

_____

Setup requirements (where you sat, where your parent sat, type of chairs used, table covering, lighting, any necessary equipment used):

_____

_____

_____

Time of day the activity was done (morning, afternoon, before or after a meal):

_____

Length of time spent at the activity:

_____

Was the activity successful? Did your parent like doing it? Did you?

_____

_____

Did you have to tweak the activity to make it work better for you or your parent? If so, describe how:

_____

_____

Did you teach another person how to do this activity, ensuring you weren't the only one to do it? If so, who?

_____

Would you do this activity again? Yes or no? Why or why not

_____

_____

_____

Going to the Market

I like going to the grocery store with my mother. It is a familiar task she has done for years. What makes it a good activity for someone with dementia is that it requires a plan. Prior to leaving for the market, you have to assess what it is you need to purchase. You must create a list. Afterward you can search for corresponding coupons. Then you are ready to go.

The market can provide overwhelming stimulation. The colors, noises, lights, and smells might be too much for those individuals struggling with moderate to late-stage dementia but not necessarily for those in the mild to moderate level. Determine which size market works best for your parent. Just because you might have shopped at a huge super store in the past doesn't mean it remains appropriate now. The small corner market can offer individual contact and personal service amid calmer and less visually arousing surroundings.

My mother likes to push the shopping cart. This task gives her something substantial to hold. It also seems to "ground" her within the market, helping her feel oriented and productive. When we arrive at the desired shelf, we refer back to our coupons. The picture of the product helps my mother locate the desired item. While shopping, we discuss different foods we see, and sometimes we choose a new item to try.

Once you are home, have your parent fold the grocery bags after you empty them.

Shopping at the market can provide a full morning of functional activity with a satisfying ending. After all, who doesn't like to eat?

Assess This Activity

Date: _____

Name of activity:

_____

Setup location (inside, outside, at a table, in which room):

_____

Setup requirements (where you sat, where your parent sat, type of chairs used, table covering, lighting, any necessary equipment used):

_____

_____

_____

Time of day the activity was done (morning, afternoon, before or after a meal):

_____

Length of time spent at the activity:

_____

Was the activity successful? Did your parent like doing it? Did you?

_____

_____

Did you have to tweak the activity to make it work better for you or your parent? If so, describe how:

_____

_____

Did you teach another person how to do this activity, ensuring you weren't the only one to do it? If so, who?

_____

Would you do this activity again? Yes or no? Why or why not

_____

_____

_____

Having a Conversation

Sometimes you don't need to do an activity or task with your parent per se; you just need to visit. There's no activity to arrange or set up. There's no consideration about the correct lighting, about where you are seated, or about whether you have everything positioned "just so." Relax and have a conversation with your parent. Sounds so simple...and it is. Just sit down, have a cup of tea or coffee, and chat with your parent about anything that comes to mind: a recent vacation you might have taken, your child's new job, your grandchildren's school progress, or their little league accomplishments. Any topic is fine. Ask your parent about his or her siblings or about a special event he or she remembers from when he or she was a child.

Often with the busyness of caring for your parent, it can be easy to forget he or she isn't just a responsibility but is still your parent. He or she is still interested in you. His or her participation in a conversation just might surprise you.

Assess This Activity

Date: _____

Name of activity:

_____

Setup location (inside, outside, at a table, in which room):

_____

Setup requirements (where you sat, where your parent sat, type of chairs used, table covering, lighting, any necessary equipment used):

_____

_____

_____

Time of day the activity was done (morning, afternoon, before or after a meal):

_____

Length of time spent at the activity:

_____

Was the activity successful? Did your parent like doing it? Did you?

_____

_____

Did you have to tweak the activity to make it work better for you or your parent? If so, describe how:

_____

_____

Did you teach another person how to do this activity, ensuring you weren't the only one to do it? If so, who?

_____

Would you do this activity again? Yes or no? Why or why not

_____

_____

_____

LAUNDRY DAY

The need to do laundry is a given. Someone is always making something dirty. So what better task than to get it clean and make it an activity to do with your parent in the process? What may be a boring and repetitive routine for you can remain interesting and satisfying for him or her.

I have found that multiple-step instructions are often confusing. Instead I try to give clear one-step requests. Be specific. Begin by explaining your plans and telling your parent how he or she will be included in the task. For example, "Today is Tuesday, and we are going to do the laundry. Would you help me empty out the hamper?" When that step is completed, you can further add, "Would you help me separate the laundry into piles of colored clothes and white clothes?"

Once the laundry is sorted, carrying it to the washer and putting it into the machine are the next steps. Your parent can help measure the detergent. If this step is too difficult, you can measure the amount, and he or she can pour it in. Then set the timer and ask him or her to listen for the bell indicating that the load is finished. You might have to periodically remind him or her to listen for it as well as to explain "why." Next have him or her put the wet clothes into the dryer. As before, instruct your parent to listen for the timer indicating that the clothes are dry. And again, you might have to remind him or her more than once to listen for the bell.

When all the clothes are clean, you are on to sorting by item, folding, matching socks into pairs, and then putting all the clean laundry away into appropriate drawers.

Assess This Activity

Date: _____

Name of activity:

_____

Setup location (inside, outside, at a table, in which room):

_____

Setup requirements (where you sat, where your parent sat, type of chairs used, table covering, lighting, any necessary equipment used):

_____

_____

_____

Time of day the activity was done (morning, afternoon, before or after a meal):

_____

Length of time spent at the activity:

_____

Was the activity successful? Did your parent like doing it? Did you?

_____

_____

Did you have to tweak the activity to make it work better for you or your parent? If so, describe how:

_____

_____

Did you teach another person how to do this activity, ensuring you weren't the only one to do it? If so, who?

_____

Would you do this activity again? Yes or no? Why or why not

_____

_____

_____

LETTER TILES

Personally, I like word board games. I like the challenge of creating words and scoring points. My mother continues to love word games. She had a background in Latin that served her well all these years, and her familiarity with words made her a true word champion.

With the onset of her dementia, I have found another use for the tiles. Because they are usually made from wood, they are substantial in texture, and the letters printed on them are easily visible.

I have come up with an abundance of letter tile activities for my activity arsenal. My mother and I sit together at a well-lit table I have covered with a light-colored cloth or towel. Then I pour all the tiles onto the cloth. My mother turns all the tiles so the printed side faces upward. We then sort them by consonant or vowel, followed by arranging each letter into a vertical row. We can then check to see which row is the longest to determine which letter appears the most frequently. We count them as a double check and write down the number on a nearby piece of paper. When we are finished with this activity, we add the numbers to see how many tiles we have altogether.

We have also arranged the tiles in alphabetical order. We have spelled our names and specific words with them. We have formed them into shapes, and we have stacked them in towers. We have challenged each other to see who could build the tallest tower before it fell over.

When we reach the end of our tolerance for letter tiles, we collect them alphabetically and return them to the container.

Assess This Activity

Date: _____

Name of activity:

_____

Setup location (inside, outside, at a table, in which room):

_____

Setup requirements (where you sat, where your parent sat, type of chairs used, table covering, lighting, any necessary equipment used):

_____

_____

_____

Time of day the activity was done (morning, afternoon, before or after a meal):

_____

Length of time spent at the activity:

_____

Was the activity successful? Did your parent like doing it? Did you?

_____

_____

Did you have to tweak the activity to make it work better for you or your parent? If so, describe how:

_____

_____

Did you teach another person how to do this activity, ensuring you weren't the only one to do it? If so, who?

_____

Would you do this activity again? Yes or no? Why or why not

_____

_____

_____

Mah Jongg

Mah Jongg is a social game played with tiles. My mother was part of a group of women with whom she played this game once a week. This group met for more than fifty years, and these friends had a great time being together. Now just seeing the tiles evokes the best of memories for her.

The tiles in a Mah Jongg set are beautiful. The older tiles can be made from ivory, from Bakelite, or most recently from plastic. The designs on them are flowers and different suits (similar to playing cards) called "cracks, bams, and dots," and most of the tiles are numbered. The colors are bright and clear. The tiles are substantive to hold and are easy to keep clean. I love these tiles!

Needless to say, my mother can no longer play the game, but the tiles are just great to use for building and making designs. Nowhere is it written that you have to use something in the same way forever.

Similarly to how we use dominoes, we use Mah Jongg tiles to build towers and see how high we can get before they fall over. We turn them all faceup or facedown. We sort them by suit. We count them. We create letters from them. We make designs by laying them flat, and we create interest by turning some of them on their sides. We are limited only by our imaginations.

Mah Jongg sets can be found on eBay. You can purchase just the tiles without the rest of the game by e-mailing the National Mah Jongg League.

Assess This Activity

Date: _____

Name of activity:

_____

Setup location (inside, outside, at a table, in which room):

_____

Setup requirements (where you sat, where your parent sat, type of chairs used, table covering, lighting, any necessary equipment used):

_____

_____

_____

Time of day the activity was done (morning, afternoon, before or after a meal):

_____

Length of time spent at the activity:

_____

Was the activity successful? Did your parent like doing it? Did you?

_____

_____

Did you have to tweak the activity to make it work better for you or your parent? If so, describe how:

_____

_____

Did you teach another person how to do this activity, ensuring you weren't the only one to do it? If so, who?

_____

Would you do this activity again? Yes or no? Why or why not

_____

_____

_____

MAKING A CALENDAR

With the onset of dementia, my mother has lost the concept of time. She's not sure what year it is, let alone the month or day of the week. The benefit of a large, visible calendar is that it structures time and reminds her of what she will be doing and when.

Twelve pieces of paper, a ruler, and a pen are all you need to get started making your own calendar. Follow the familiar format with the paper placed horizontally and leave space at the top for writing in the month. Below it make a grid of squares each approximately two and a half inches in size. You will need seven squares across and five rows down to account for all the dates in the varying months.

If your parent is able, he or she can draw the calendar grid. If not, you can draw the grid in pencil and have him or her draw over your lines with a dark marker. If your parent is still unable, you can draw the grid and have it ready for him or her to begin filling in the months, the days of the week, and the dates for the days in the squares. Or simply buy a large, plain office calendar. Choose one that doesn't add preprinted events or designs, which can be both distracting and confusing.

This activity promotes the ability to sequence (for example, months of the year, days of the week, counting from one to thirty-one days). Because of the repetition necessary to complete multiple months, the activity becomes easier as you progress. If your parent gets frustrated, you have natural stopping points as you finish each week or month.

I like this activity a lot. It's functional and useful. While working on our calendar, my mother and I listed the four different seasons and discussed the type of weather found at that time. Is it hot? Is it cold? Will she need a jacket? What other type of clothing might be worn during that season? We have entered holidays and birthdays, and even listed scheduled medical appointments. We cross off the days as they pass.

Assess This Activity

Name of activity:

_____

Setup location (inside, outside, at a table, in which room):

_____

Setup requirements (where you sat, where your parent sat, type of chairs used, table covering, lighting, any necessary equipment used):

_____

_____

_____

Time of day the activity was done (morning, afternoon, before or after a meal):

_____

Length of time spent at the activity:

_____

Was the activity successful? Did your parent like doing it? Did you?

_____

_____

Did you have to tweak the activity to make it work better for you or your parent? If so, describe how:

_____

_____

Did you teach another person how to do this activity, ensuring you weren't the only one to do it? If so, who?

_____

Would you do this activity again? Yes or no? Why or why not

_____

_____

_____

Making a Clock

ime, as well as the concept of time, can be confusing for those with dementia. There is no day of the week, no month, and no year. Everything is the same. The idea of daytime versus nighttime can be lost along with memory. That doesn't mean there cannot be structure or that you shouldn't try to reinforce one. The goal is to create a framework that is meaningful for your parent.

The task of making a clock is an activity that targets shapes (circles), counting, sequencing, and hopefully a structure that can be used to start and close any task.

If able, have your parent draw or trace a ten- to twelve-inch circle for the face of the clock. You can use a dinner plate as your template. Then have him or her cut the face out. You can do these steps for your parent if he or she is unable.

I prefer that my mother not draw the numbers directly on the clock face. If she should put them in the wrong place, we would have to begin again. Instead, on small one-inch squares of paper I have my mother write a number on each—one through twelve. Then we begin the placement of the hours, starting with number twelve at the top. We discuss where the bottom of the circle is located and place the number six there. We continue with the three and then the nine before proceeding with the other numbers. We then tape them into place. I make the hands for the clock and attach them to the center of the clock with a brass tack.

Then we get to work. We review the concepts of "morning," "afternoon," and "evening." After looking at the calendar, we discuss our plans for that morning. We figure out what time an event will take place, and we make the time on the clock correspond. We talk about what we will do "first" and what will happen "after" that specific time. We also discuss how much time needs to pass before that event arrives and what we have to do to get ready.

Assess This Activity

Date: _____

Name of activity:

_____

Setup location (inside, outside, at a table, in which room):

_____

Setup requirements (where you sat, where your parent sat, type of chairs used, table covering, lighting, any necessary equipment used):

_____

_____

_____

Time of day the activity was done (morning, afternoon, before or after a meal):

_____

Length of time spent at the activity:

_____

Was the activity successful? Did your parent like doing it? Did you?

_____

_____

Did you have to tweak the activity to make it work better for you or your parent? If so, describe how:

_____

_____

Did you teach another person how to do this activity, ensuring you weren't the only one to do it? If so, who?

_____

Would you do this activity again? Yes or no? Why or why not

_____

_____

_____

MATCHING GAMES

atching items can be enjoyable. Employing familiar objects found around the house, we have been able to match by color, shape, use, feel, and smell. I try not to use more than three to four objects at a time since they can get too confusing.

When choosing color matching as our activity, I select from my ever-growing collection of crayons, pop-it beads, spools of thread, as well as fruits, both real and fake in photographs. I have often used grapes, oranges, and apples. Then I have my mother put all the red objects (for example, an apple, a crayon, or a spool of thread) into one pile, all the orange objects into another pile, and so on until all are used. We then discuss what each color is and talk about which color she likes best. Frequently, our discussion goes off on a tangent. That is fine too.

My mother has an abundance of gloves and socks. I present them mixed together and have her sort them into two piles. Once they are separated, we further sort them by pattern and color. We discuss where on the body each is used.

We have matched objects by shape and size. I have used my trusty buttons, pot lids, and coins for circles; and playing cards, envelopes, and cereal boxes for rectangles. I mix them all together, and then we separate them by shape. I follow the same format as before.

Other objects easily available for sorting are found in the kitchen. Everyone has silverware. I give my mother all the forks, spoons, and knives. I leave one of each in the drawer compartments to indicate where they should be placed. She must then put the utensils back into the proper compartment. We discuss what each is used for and what we like best to eat.

Sometimes I wonder if I'm being silly, but each activity offers me a starting point for conversation, offers time together, and is something satisfying for her to do.

Assess This Activity

Date: _____

Name of activity:

_____

Setup location (inside, outside, at a table, in which room):

_____

Setup requirements (where you sat, where your parent sat, type of chairs used, table covering, lighting, any necessary equipment used):

_____

_____

_____

Time of day the activity was done (morning, afternoon, before or after a meal):

_____

Length of time spent at the activity:

_____

Was the activity successful? Did your parent like doing it? Did you?

_____

_____

Did you have to tweak the activity to make it work better for you or your parent? If so, describe how:

_____

_____

Did you teach another person how to do this activity, ensuring you weren't the only one to do it? If so, who?

_____

Would you do this activity again? Yes or no? Why or why not

_____

_____

_____

MEMORY GAMES

Simple memory games can be beneficial for a person with dementia. They reinforce concentration. You do have to be careful, however, because they might cause frustration. If so, you should stop and adjust the difficulty level or change to an altogether different activity, so be prepared. Sometimes my mother is able to excel at this, and some days she just can't. Since there's no way to tell what type of day it will be, it's something I try. If it interests her, I continue. If not, I move on.

One memory game I often play is a take-away game. I place three objects on the table. I have used a spoon, a cup, and a pencil. I name the objects and then ask her to repeat the names. I ask her to close her eyes while I remove one of the objects. Then after she reopens her eyes, she has to tell me which one is missing. Initially when we played this game, I was able to include more objects. As she has lost cognitive ability, I have used fewer.

Another game I have chosen uses playing cards. Using a total of eight cards, I select pairs that match by color and number. I try to decrease confusion by selecting only cards with numbers and pictures that look different from each other. An example is two cards with red kings, two cards with the number three in black, two cards with the number ten in red, and so forth. Then I mix the cards together and turn them facedown to form a grid. We alternate turning over two cards at a time. If they match, they become the win pile. If not, we return them to the facedown position, and the next player takes his or her turn. If this is too difficult, I decrease the number of paired cards being used.

One last game I have used incorporates memory with tactile discrimination. With her eyes closed, I place a familiar object into her hands. The object has to be large enough with specific distinguishing characteristics that she will be able to figure it out. She has to describe what she is feeling and then name it. I make sure to choose only items she continues to use on a daily basis. Examples of items I have used include a hairbrush, fork, spoon, ball, and comb.

Assess This Activity

Date: _____

Name of activity:

Setup location (inside, outside, at a table, in which room):

Setup requirements (where you sat, where your parent sat, type of chairs used, table covering, lighting, any necessary equipment used):

Time of day the activity was done (morning, afternoon, before or after a meal):

Length of time spent at the activity:

Was the activity successful? Did your parent like doing it? Did you?

Did you have to tweak the activity to make it work better for you or your parent? If so, describe how:

Did you teach another person how to do this activity, ensuring you weren't the only one to do it? If so, who?

Would you do this activity again? Yes or no? Why or why not

MONEY AND COINS

Paper money and coins are familiar objects. Your parents have used these for their purchases their entire lifetimes. The use of money, counting, and the simple math it requires was part of their daily routines. The concept of a dollar and its equivalent amounts in quarters, dimes, nickels, and pennies is something most people can remember even if they have dementia.

Place a towel over your table so no coins roll off and pour out the change from your bank. You can have your parent sort the coins by denomination. You can place them in rows by size order. Discuss which coins are physically larger, which are smaller, which coins are silver or copper in color. Count them to determine the total amount. I like to discuss which coin is worth the most. I also like to make equivalents—for example, a dollar equals four quarters, a nickel equals five pennies, and so forth.

I have given my mother simple addition tasks to do with coins. For example, I have asked her to give me twelve cents or eighty-three cents. I try to ask for an amount that requires more than one type of coin. She has to find the coins that add up to that amount. I have also asked her subtraction questions. For example, when she has twelve cents and she gives me a nickel, how much does she have left? What was once routine is now difficult.

We have used the coins to make designs, such as faces or flowers. We have each taken a handful of coins and lined them up in rows. We count which row has the highest monetary value.

We have stacked the coins to see how high we can go before they fall over. We have played games in which we hold the coins in our hands and place them one by one into the bank, making sure not to drop any. Finally, we have played games in which we close our eyes and have to guess which coin we are holding based on feel alone.

Our activities are limited only by our imaginations.

Assess This Activity

Date: _____

Name of activity:

_____

Setup location (inside, outside, at a table, in which room):

_____

Setup requirements (where you sat, where your parent sat, type of chairs used, table covering, lighting, any necessary equipment used):

_____

_____

_____

Time of day the activity was done (morning, afternoon, before or after a meal):

_____

Length of time spent at the activity:

_____

Was the activity successful? Did your parent like doing it? Did you?

_____

_____

Did you have to tweak the activity to make it work better for you or your parent? If so, describe how:

_____

_____

Did you teach another person how to do this activity, ensuring you weren't the only one to do it? If so, who?

_____

Would you do this activity again? Yes or no? Why or why not

_____

_____

_____

Music

All people love music, especially songs they knew when they were young. That is the music that is familiar and memorable. In my mother's case, she recalls the music of the 1940s. Often she can't retrieve something said to her only moments before, yet she is capable of singing every word to songs from World War II—and they played on the radio seventy to eighty years earlier! Music is a "memory trigger". It leads to recollections of events that occurred around the same time as a specific song.

For her birthday this year, I bought my mother an AM/FM/CD player with disks of music from the 1940s. This was the big band era with Benny Goodman, Frank Sinatra, the Andrews Sisters—music that has a swing beat. The music places her back in time. She loves it. She spends time singing, humming, clapping her hands, and moving her feet to the rhythm of the songs.

Conversely, I have also found that this same music can quiet her. At times, when she walks from room to room, looking for something "missing," we turn on the music. When it begins, she gets calmer. She then sits on the sofa and simply listens.

The respite the music provides gives her caretaker some time to do other housekeeping tasks. It also gives both of them a few precious minutes to themselves.

Assess This Activity

Date: _____

Name of activity:

_____

Setup location (inside, outside, at a table, in which room):

_____

Setup requirements (where you sat, where your parent sat, type of chairs used, table covering, lighting, any necessary equipment used):

_____

_____

_____

Time of day the activity was done (morning, afternoon, before or after a meal):

_____

Length of time spent at the activity:

_____

Was the activity successful? Did your parent like doing it? Did you?

_____

_____

Did you have to tweak the activity to make it work better for you or your parent? If so, describe how:

_____

_____

Did you teach another person how to do this activity, ensuring you weren't the only one to do it? If so, who?

_____

Would you do this activity again? Yes or no? Why or why not

_____

_____

_____

Musical Instruments

$\mathcal{D}$id your parent ever play an instrument? Mine didn't. Her brother always played the piano, and my children have played the guitar and cello. My mother was exposed to these instruments when she went to concerts in the past and when she watched her family play, but she never took up playing an instrument.

I thought using instruments might be something my mother would enjoy, so I purchased a kit of children's instruments from my local toy store. Included in the set is a triangle, a castanet, a kazoo, a drum with a stick, and a wrist strap with an attached bell. What a perfect collection, and it is colorful too.

All the instruments are small enough to be held in her lap. What a great activity to do from a sitting position or, if need be, from a lying position. The only caveat would be this: if your parent has breathing difficulties, I would limit or omit the use of the kazoo since it might increase shortness of breath. I found that the wrist bell was something my mother could use while either sitting or lying down. If your parent has more advanced dementia, the wrist bell might be useful for him or her since it doesn't require grasping. Once you have placed it on him or her, only arm motion is required to initiate sound.

My mother has now tested each instrument. Her decision-making skills are encouraged as she must choose the one she will use while she listens to her 1940s music. Now, in addition to her humming and singing, she has the added option of playing along as well. The caretaker and I often take part as we create our miniband at home.

Assess This Activity

Date: _____

Name of activity:

_____

Setup location (inside, outside, at a table, in which room):

_____

Setup requirements (where you sat, where your parent sat, type of chairs used, table covering, lighting, any necessary equipment used):

_____

_____

_____

Time of day the activity was done (morning, afternoon, before or after a meal):

_____

Length of time spent at the activity:

_____

Was the activity successful? Did your parent like doing it? Did you?

_____

_____

Did you have to tweak the activity to make it work better for you or your parent? If so, describe how:

_____

_____

Did you teach another person how to do this activity, ensuring you weren't the only one to do it? If so, who?

_____

Would you do this activity again? Yes or no? Why or why not

_____

_____

_____

PATTERN MATCHING

I like patterns, and my mother does as well. They are easy to make, and the concept is easy to understand. To start, you will need several different items and three to four multiple pieces of each. Create your pattern row using several different items. Place your design across the center of the table. Your parent can then copy his or her design below yours. If he or she is capable, the amount of objects used in the design may be increased.

I have used many common household articles to form my patterns. Large colored beads, dominoes, spoons, forks, pencils, playing cards, and even spools of thread have found their way into my designs. I have also asked my mother for suggestions of items she would like to employ when making her patterns. A design I once created included a row comprising a fork, a spool of thread, a domino (with the white dots facing down)—and ending with a pencil. Then, choosing the duplicates of these same items, which I had previously placed into a box, my mother copied the pattern.

I have made pattern rows from pieces of colored paper. Red, blue, yellow, green—I make my design using as many rows as my mother's cognition that day allows. And again, she copies her pattern below mine.

If your parent has the manual dexterity and vision, another way to make pattern designs is with large stringing beads. They can be found in children's toy stores. First, you create your string of four to five different-colored beads, followed by your parent copying your design onto his or her string.

You can vary this activity by having your parent initiate the design, which you then copy. With this scenario your parent has to determine whether you are correct.

The pattern designs are infinite.

Assess This Activity

Name of activity:

_____

Setup location (inside, outside, at a table, in which room):

_____

Setup requirements (where you sat, where your parent sat, type of chairs used, table covering, lighting, any necessary equipment used):

_____

_____

_____

Time of day the activity was done (morning, afternoon, before or after a meal):

_____

Length of time spent at the activity:

_____

Was the activity successful? Did your parent like doing it? Did you?

_____

_____

Did you have to tweak the activity to make it work better for you or your parent? If so, describe how:

_____

_____

Did you teach another person how to do this activity, ensuring you weren't the only one to do it? If so, who?

_____

Would you do this activity again? Yes or no? Why or why not

_____

_____

_____

PEGS AND PEGBOARDS

I love pegs and pegboards. In the past, while working as an occupational therapist, I used them for hand control, prehension skills, coordination, color discrimination, and pattern matching. Using Velcro, I attached rubber pegboards to the wall and encouraged patients to increase both their arm range of motion and arm strength as they reached upward to insert the pegs into the board. I used them with clients who'd had strokes, arm weakness, coordination problems—and also for those who had cognitive problems, such as Alzheimer's dementia. Pegs and pegboard remain a perfect tool for my arsenal.

Pegboards come in a variety of materials. Often they are made from wood, a surface that is hard, smooth, and nonresistant. The pegs are made from wood as well. Because of this lack of resistance, they are easily inserted into the holes. These pegs are straight, and the width can vary from one-quarter to one inch thick; in some cases they come in varying heights—from one inch to five inches tall. They come in multiple colors and require good hand control and vision to use.

Pegboards can also be made from rubber and are sold with large, bulbous, multicolored pegs that are often made from plastic. While their shape makes them easy to see and grip, the friction from the rubber board against these pegs requires increased effort for insertion. They require more hand strength, greater endurance, and a stronger grip—something that can be difficult for those with arthritis.

While pegs are usually made from round dowels, other shapes are available as well. I have seen square pegs as well as star-shaped pegs. These are more difficult to use since they require increased cognition to manipulate appropriately into the board; this is a limitation for those with more advanced dementia.

Usually there are one hundred pegs per board, ten rows of ten holes. Because of this large size, it is possible to make a design across the top that leaves room for your parent to make his or her design below yours across the bottom of the board. Ensure that there are enough of each colored pegs so your parent's design can match yours. For example, your design can be two blues, two reds, two yellows, and four greens across the top. Once your pattern is completed, ask your parent to choose the necessary pegs and copy your design across the bottom.

You can also put the pegs into the board by color. For example, have your parent put in all the reds, then all the greens, and so on to the end. Encourage him or her to remember what color he or she is working with by having your parent repeat it as he or she progresses. If his or her attention span is short, limit the task to completing only one row. Encourage decision making by asking him or her to select the color he or she will use.

Putting pegs into a pegboard is a good activity that is repetitive and easily understood. It can take up a good amount of time, and once you are sure your parent can follow through, it's something he or she can work with by himself or herself.

Assess This Activity

Date: _____

Name of activity:

_____

Setup location (inside, outside, at a table, in which room):

_____

Setup requirements (where you sat, where your parent sat, type of chairs used, table covering, lighting, any necessary equipment used):

_____

_____

_____

Time of day the activity was done (morning, afternoon, before or after a meal):

_____

Length of time spent at the activity:

_____

Was the activity successful? Did your parent like doing it? Did you?

_____

_____

Did you have to tweak the activity to make it work better for you or your parent? If so, describe how:

_____

_____

Did you teach another person how to do this activity, ensuring you weren't the only one to do it? If so, who?

_____

Would you do this activity again? Yes or no? Why or why not

_____

_____

_____

PETS

What could be more beneficial for someone with dementia than having a pet? The act of stroking and caring for an animal is calming. Dogs and even cats offer a source of warmth, companionship, and unconditional affection. The daily routine of walking and being with them can structure the day. You must be aware, however, that as dementia progresses, what may have once been a joy may now become a burden or even a problem for your parent.

Changes with your parent's cognition and physical status require you to revisit what type of animal he or she owns and whether it still remains appropriate for him or her. That young, rambunctious dog might be too frisky for someone with balance problems and may potentially cause falls when your parent is walking. The need to take the dog outside early in the morning in poor weather or when it is dark might be difficult for someone who has no concept of time or has decreased vision.

If you still wish to choose a new pet, consider looking for a retired therapy dog. Look on the Internet under "service dogs." There might be one available within your neighborhood. I have worked in many long-term care facilities that offer visits from therapy dogs. Perhaps visits such as these might be arranged at your parent's home and could eliminate the need for him or her to own a pet.

Your parent might move to another location where animals are not allowed. In this instance tropical fish might be the animal to consider. They provide a constant source of movement, which is comforting for those who are agitated. Choose brightly colored, large fish that are easily seen against the backdrop of the tank.

Even easier is a "virtual" fish tank. This tank, which you fill with water, comes with multi-colored plastic fish. The fish are controlled by battery and their swimming motion mimics that seen with live fish. No concern about feeding or cleaning issues with this tank. I found it on Amazon.com. It offers the benefits of continuous slow motion that real fish create without the worry and requirements of actual care.

Assess This Activity

Date: _____

Name of activity:

_____

Setup location (inside, outside, at a table, in which room):

_____

Setup requirements (where you sat, where your parent sat, type of chairs used, table covering, lighting, any necessary equipment used):

_____

_____

_____

Time of day the activity was done (morning, afternoon, before or after a meal):

_____

Length of time spent at the activity:

_____

Was the activity successful? Did your parent like doing it? Did you?

_____

_____

Did you have to tweak the activity to make it work better for you or your parent? If so, describe how:

_____

_____

Did you teach another person how to do this activity, ensuring you weren't the only one to do it? If so, who?

_____

Would you do this activity again? Yes or no? Why or why not

_____

_____

_____

Photo Albums

y mother has albums of photos taken during family events and past celebrations. We have spent many hours going through them. She can still remember the faces of her friends and, with some prompting from me, can recall their names. I have written names and captions under the photographs to further describe the images. This step provides a helpful tool for the caregiver when I'm unavailable. These images and stories bring a smile to her face and help stimulate conversations. I'm careful not to mention whether someone in the photograph has died.

We have reviewed my wedding album. She can pick out the bride (me) since I'm the one wearing the white dress. She can find herself if I give her a hint as to what she was wearing. She loves looking at pictures of herself with my father, especially those in which they are dancing.

I have also been able to locate some pictures of my mother when she was a child, though there aren't many of these. Inevitably this leads to discussions about her parents, and each time she tells me what a beautiful woman her mother was.

While the albums recall the past, I'm also interested in helping her retain the present. In an attempt to have my mother remember my family, I have placed a grouping of their photographs on her kitchen table. Because of her decreased vision, I have made sure all the pictures are large and of only their faces. On white cards I have used a black marker to write down each of the corresponding names. Initially we made a game of matching the names to the pictures. Now the names are taped to the pictures, and we just read and point to each, naming something special about each person.

Assess This Activity

Date: _____

Name of activity:

_____

Setup location (inside, outside, at a table, in which room):

_____

Setup requirements (where you sat, where your parent sat, type of chairs used, table covering, lighting, any necessary equipment used):

_____

_____

_____

Time of day the activity was done (morning, afternoon, before or after a meal):

_____

Length of time spent at the activity:

_____

Was the activity successful? Did your parent like doing it? Did you?

_____

_____

Did you have to tweak the activity to make it work better for you or your parent? If so, describe how:

_____

_____

Did you teach another person how to do this activity, ensuring you weren't the only one to do it? If so, who?

_____

Would you do this activity again? Yes or no? Why or why not

_____

_____

_____

Playing Cards

I enjoy cards. I like their colors and the clarity of the numbers. I like that they have a design on the back that is different from that on the face. I like their tactile input and appreciate the hand coordination necessary to shuffle them together. Primarily, I like that they are familiar and something most people have played with in the past.

Cards and card games require memory and attention to the rules as well as focus on the cards themselves. Playing a card game also encourages decision making. I encourage my mother to decide which task she would like to do. I also encourage her to determine when she has had enough and wants to stop.

There are so many activities to do with a deck of cards. They can be counted and divided into two, three, or four piles. They can be sorted by suit. They can be arranged by suits in ascending order from ace or one up to king. At times I have mixed up all the cards and had my mother locate all four of a specific number. This activity specifically targets memory skills since she has to remember the number I requested. I have also mixed the cards faceup and facedown, and asked her to readjust them so all are placed in the same direction.

My mother was a great bridge player, and she still has "card sense." She enjoys any game with cards. We have always played gin rummy. At this time she no longer recognizes the name *gin,* yet she is still able to play the game. As soon as I deal out the cards, she knows just what to do. She still wins.

The game we now most frequently play is War. The concept of a greater-versus-smaller number is something she still comprehends. What is also convenient about this game is that we can stop at any time should either of us decide to quit. We simply count the cards to see who won.

There are many decks of cards around our house, and no two decks have the same design on the back. As another activity, I often mix two different-patterned decks together and have her separate them.

When we are finished with any of these activities, we count the completed decks to make sure they each have the requisite fifty-two cards before putting them away.

Assess This Activity

Date: _____

Name of activity:

_____

Setup location (inside, outside, at a table, in which room):

_____

Setup requirements (where you sat, where your parent sat, type of chairs used, table covering, lighting, any necessary equipment used):

_____

_____

_____

Time of day the activity was done (morning, afternoon, before or after a meal):

_____

Length of time spent at the activity:

_____

Was the activity successful? Did your parent like doing it? Did you?

_____

_____

Did you have to tweak the activity to make it work better for you or your parent? If so, describe how:

_____

_____

Did you teach another person how to do this activity, ensuring you weren't the only one to do it? If so, who?

_____

Would you do this activity again? Yes or no? Why or why not

_____

_____

_____

Playing Catch

Catch is a great exercise. It can target standing balance and tolerance, eye-hand coordination, and reflex response time. It also provides upper-body activity and mobility.

Catch can be played from either a standing or a sitting position. If you choose standing, place a chair nearby in case of fatigue. Take into consideration your parent's balance and whether he or she can lift his or her arms into the air without falling to the side. His or her feet should be solidly planted shoulder width apart, and shoes should be flat soled. Should he or she begin to sway or get breathless, that is your cue to have him or her do the activity while sitting.

Before you toss the ball, give verbal prompts. Examples might be "Get ready" or "I'm going to toss it to you now." Don't assume he or she knows the ball is coming; your parent probably hasn't done this in decades. Consider bouncing instead of throwing the ball to him or her. This tip provides more time to prepare and makes catching easier. If you opt to play catch from a seated position again, don't forget to give the prompts that the ball is coming.

The ball I prefer to use is a large twelve-inch to four-teen-inch beach ball. I have even used a large balloon. I find each to be light, easy to see, and easy to catch. This size necessitates use of the arms in addition to the hands. The balloon moves more slowly through the air and therefore is easier to catch than the beach ball. This is the better choice if your parent's reflexes or vision has decreased.

I get bored using activities the same way, therefore I also vary how we play. When seated at the table, instead of tossing the ball, we roll it across the table to each other. To make this even more structured, I have formed two parallel lines across the tabletop that are approximately sixteen inches apart. They are created from rolled-up towels, dominoes, or even playing cards. When we roll the ball, it has to remain between the two lines all the way across the tabletop before we catch it.

Assess This Activity

Date: _____

Name of activity:

_____

Setup location (inside, outside, at a table, in which room):

_____

Setup requirements (where you sat, where your parent sat, type of chairs used, table covering, lighting, any necessary equipment used):

_____

_____

_____

Time of day the activity was done (morning, afternoon, before or after a meal):

_____

Length of time spent at the activity:

_____

Was the activity successful? Did your parent like doing it? Did you?

_____

_____

Did you have to tweak the activity to make it work better for you or your parent? If so, describe how:

_____

_____

Did you teach another person how to do this activity, ensuring you weren't the only one to do it? If so, who?

_____

Would you do this activity again? Yes or no? Why or why not

_____

_____

_____

POP-IT BEADS

An object that is easy to find in a local toy store or even in the supermarket is pop-it beads. I like them because they are large, are easy to hold, are easy to clean, and come in bold colors. A fantastic find!

My mother and I have done several activities with these beads. We have taken them apart and put them back together again. We have sorted them by color. We have counted them to determine which color has the greatest amount. We have lined them up in rows from the largest amount to the fewest.

Don't assume your parent knows how to attach them together. Take time to explain how they work. They can then be assembled by a specific color chosen by either you or your parent. A more difficult way to reattach them is by alternating colors to ensure no two of the same color beads are touching. The activity sounds easy, but that's not always so. It depends on your parent's level of cognition.

The beads can be attached to form a circle, which we have then placed flat on the tabletop. We follow this activity with a discussion of it's relationship to the placement of other objects. My mother, with directions from me, has placed items inside, above, below, and to the right and left of the pop-it bead circle. This past week we used the pop–it bead circle as a hoop. She determined the number of times she would throw a beach ball through the hoop, then counted as she did so. She was able to maintain the count and knew when she had finished. She was the one to determine she had done enough.

When you are finished with the beads, you can take them apart and again sort them by color or quantity—greatest or smallest. Then return them to the storage container using the same sorting method as before.

Assess This Activity

Date: _____

Name of activity:

_____

Setup location (inside, outside, at a table, in which room):

_____

Setup requirements (where you sat, where your parent sat, type of chairs used, table covering, lighting, any necessary equipment used):

_____

_____

_____

Time of day the activity was done (morning, afternoon, before or after a meal):

_____

Length of time spent at the activity:

_____

Was the activity successful? Did your parent like doing it? Did you?

_____

_____

Did you have to tweak the activity to make it work better for you or your parent? If so, describe how:

_____

_____

Did you teach another person how to do this activity, ensuring you weren't the only one to do it? If so, who?

_____

Would you do this activity again? Yes or no? Why or why not

_____

_____

_____

Puzzles

I love puzzles; my mother does as well. Just make sure to match the quantity of pieces to the level your parent is able to complete. Start with the count you think he or she can handle. You will know when to decrease that number when and if the puzzle becomes too frustrating or difficult for him or her. Choose a design that's simple with clear, large sections of one color that are easy to match. A single picture is best, one that isn't juvenile.

Keep the picture on the puzzle box in view to remember the goal and refer to it while you are working. Begin by separating the straight-edged border pieces from the inside irregular ones. Return those you're not using back into the box. You can start by forming the border or by matching a large block of color.

Initially my mother was able to work twenty-four piece puzzles. As time passed, I had to decrease the amount down to two-piece puzzles. I have found puzzles of animals that require matching the animal to the first letter of its name as well as a puzzle requiring her to match the animal's head with its tail. We have had many discussions about the animals. Are they wild or tame? What kind of climate do they live in? My mother was able to match pieces based on animals with striped tails, birds, those with solid-colored bodies, spotted bodies, and the type of animal that might be tame enough to be a pet. This organization led to discussions about pets she had while growing up.

At this time I use one-piece wooden shape puzzles. The colors they come in are vivid and easily seen. Because they are made from wood, they are rigid and offer another form of tactile stimulation. We discuss the colors and spend time coming up with everyday objects that match that shape. For example, a yellow circle piece reminds her of the sun. She can also name flowers or foods that are yellow. She has remained interested, and the activity holds her attention.

Assess This Activity

Name of activity:

_____

Setup location (inside, outside, at a table, in which room):

_____

Setup requirements (where you sat, where your parent sat, type of chairs used, table covering, lighting, any necessary equipment used):

_____

_____

_____

Time of day the activity was done (morning, afternoon, before or after a meal):

_____

Length of time spent at the activity:

_____

Was the activity successful? Did your parent like doing it? Did you?

_____

_____

Did you have to tweak the activity to make it work better for you or your parent? If so, describe how:

_____

_____

Did you teach another person how to do this activity, ensuring you weren't the only one to do it? If so, who?

_____

Would you do this activity again? Yes or no? Why or why not

_____

_____

_____

Reading Aloud

Often when you are caught up with the daily necessities of caretaking, it is difficult to remember to take time out for the joy of reading. This is one way to remember happy or even sad events and to find a segue for discussion.

You can take a trip to the local library to choose a book or magazine. If that becomes too overwhelming, you can choose from articles in the daily newspaper or personal journals or even from captions in old personal photo albums. Reading aloud is a social experience. It is interactive. This isn't reading for reading's sake; rather it is a way to offer topics to explore and provides an opportunity for your parent to recall the past and reinforce the present.

If your parent is capable, have him or her read to you; if he or she cannot, you can read to him or her. Ask clear leading questions that require a response other than a mere yes or no. Make him or her think about the context of the story. Relate it to the event taking place. Relate it to the "why" of the event. Discuss the fashions worn in the pictures. Ask if he or she ever dressed like that. Relate the conversation to him or her.

Sometimes it's nice to just sit and have a conversation, and reading can be the stimulus to begin. Have a cup of coffee and a snack. Put your feet up. Relax. Get started.

Assess This Activity

Date: _____

Name of activity:

_____

Setup location (inside, outside, at a table, in which room):

_____

Setup requirements (where you sat, where your parent sat, type of chairs used, table covering, lighting, any necessary equipment used):

_____

_____

_____

Time of day the activity was done (morning, afternoon, before or after a meal):

_____

Length of time spent at the activity:

_____

Was the activity successful? Did your parent like doing it? Did you?

_____

_____

Did you have to tweak the activity to make it work better for you or your parent? If so, describe how:

_____

_____

Did you teach another person how to do this activity, ensuring you weren't the only one to do it? If so, who?

_____

Would you do this activity again? Yes or no? Why or why not

_____

_____

_____

Rice Games

Uncooked rice feels good in your hands. It is soft and smooth and has a pleasant smell. It is clean, inexpensive, and wonderful for tactile stimulation. Grabbing and releasing handfuls of rice allow you to get your hands moving without dealing with the resistance and grit of using sand or the wrinkling of skin caused by using water. It is especially good for people with arthritic hands.

I have invested in a five-pound bag of rice to use for activities with my mother. Select a large pot or small wastebasket that will be designated for just this use. Then pour in the entire bag.

A good tactile game is the following: Making sure to have duplicates of all the items, hide one of each item in the container of rice. Retain its duplicate on the tabletop. For example, I have hidden a spoon, a large button, a domino, and a wooden puzzle piece. I point to one of the duplicate items from the table and ask my mother to use just her sense of touch to locate its mate from within the rice. Once she has found and removed the duplicate from the rice bowl, she must then place it on the table next to its match. Should she select an incorrect object, it must be returned. When all of the pairs have been reassembled, she knows the task has been completed. Initially we played with three to four objects, but as my mother has lost cognition, I have reduced the quantity and ensured we use only the larger objects.

To make this activity easier, eliminate the matching component of the above task. Simply hide multiple items in the rice. Your parent has to use his or her sense of touch to find and retrieve them. Make sure you know the items you have hidden as well as the quantity of each item used so you'll know when you've retrieved them all.

Assess This Activity

Date: _____

Name of activity:

_____

Setup location (inside, outside, at a table, in which room):

_____

Setup requirements (where you sat, where your parent sat, type of chairs
used, table covering, lighting, any necessary equipment used):

_____

_____

_____

Time of day the activity was done (morning, afternoon, before or after a meal):

_____

Length of time spent at the activity:

_____

Was the activity successful? Did your parent like doing it? Did you?

_____

_____

Did you have to tweak the activity to make it work better for you or your
parent? If so, describe how:

_____

_____

Did you teach another person how to do this activity, ensuring you
weren't the only one to do it? If so, who?

_____

Would you do this activity again? Yes or no? Why or why not

_____

_____

_____

Scissors Skills and Cutting

*I*f your parent has good vision and hand coordination, using scissors to cut out pictures is an activity that might be appropriate. You can make scrapbooks from store brochures or magazines. Each page you create can be devoted to a different subject. Ask your parent to help select the topic. Subjects might include pictures of flowers, babies, or even household items. The list is endless. It can be an activity just trying to find appropriate pictures.

I tried this activity with my mother in the past, and she was able to complete it. Lately, however, she is too frustrated with the scissors, and I have taken over this part. At this time, instead of cutting out pictures of objects, I have cut out capital letters. The ones I have chosen are in different colors, fonts, and sizes. Some letters are duplicates as well. I spread the letters on the tabletop and have her put them in alphabetical order. She then has to name an object that begins with each letter.

Remember that even the best-laid plans for an activity might need to be changed. The ability to complete a task depends on the individual. Often skills on Monday can change by Tuesday. Frustration levels can also vary based on the time of day. The purpose of an activity is to help you spend your time successfully with your parent. If something doesn't catch his or her interest, move on to something else.

Assess This Activity

Date: _____

Name of activity:

_____

Setup location (inside, outside, at a table, in which room):

_____

Setup requirements (where you sat, where your parent sat, type of chairs used, table covering, lighting, any necessary equipment used):

_____

_____

_____

Time of day the activity was done (morning, afternoon, before or after a meal):

_____

Length of time spent at the activity:

_____

Was the activity successful? Did your parent like doing it? Did you?

_____

_____

Did you have to tweak the activity to make it work better for you or your parent? If so, describe how:

_____

_____

Did you teach another person how to do this activity, ensuring you weren't the only one to do it? If so, who?

_____

Would you do this activity again? Yes or no? Why or why not

_____

_____

_____

Self-Care Activities and Stress

*I*t is a blessing to have your parent perform as much as he or she can for himself or herself for as long as he or she can. This is what we all wish. It is stressful to be the one taking care of your parent and attending to his or her physical needs; this is not the way it is supposed to be.

Dementia, especially in the latter stages of the disease, can affect your parent's ability to feed, dress, wash, and bathe independently. He or she might now require assistance from you to get clean and dressed on a daily basis. This need might be stressful for him or her as well as for you.

Consider whether you're adding to your parent's stress level by how you present yourself while doing these daily activities. Step back and take a look at yourself. Do you raise your voice? Consider lowering the volume when you speak with him or her. Do you get rough when you wash or dry him or her? Consider how you would feel if a family member had to care for you. Do you resent doing these tasks for your parent?

Consider having someone else come by in the mornings to help you. Perhaps you can rotate these responsibilities with other family members. Your parent might be eligible for assistance through Medicare, Medicaid, or even through a church program. You should try to find out. Consider going to a caregiver support group in your area. You might be surprised to find that many other people are dealing with similar issues. They can be your best contacts for local resources and help.

Some activities may help decrease anxiety and stress levels, and lessen the feelings of helplessness that often accompany dementia. They allow your parent to just "feel good." You might feel good being able to offer them. Some of these activities include placing a cool compress on your parent's forehead, while he or she lies back and listens to soft and familiar music; giving him or her a back rub; combing his or her hair; rubbing in hand lotion; doing deep-breathing exercises; and stretching and giving a manicure. Also consider turning down the lights in the room and just trying to have some quiet time.

Assess This Activity

Name of activity:

_____

Setup location (inside, outside, at a table, in which room):

_____

Setup requirements (where you sat, where your parent sat, type of chairs used, table covering, lighting, any necessary equipment used):

_____

_____

_____

Time of day the activity was done (morning, afternoon, before or after a meal):

_____

Length of time spent at the activity:

_____

Was the activity successful? Did your parent like doing it? Did you?

_____

_____

Did you have to tweak the activity to make it work better for you or your parent? If so, describe how:

_____

_____

Did you teach another person how to do this activity, ensuring you weren't the only one to do it? If so, who?

_____

Would you do this activity again? Yes or no? Why or why not

_____

_____

_____

Sequencing Tasks

Sequencing tasks require you to do an activity in the proper order until completion. This activity can be difficult for someone with dementia and might require more assistance on your part.

One specific task we used both in the past when my mother was sharper and now when she requires more hints is getting her clothes ready for the next day. We describe what the weather will be like—does she have to dress for cold or warm weather?—and then we begin. I ask her to retrieve the clothing in the order in which she would put it on, starting with her underwear and progressing to her sweater. Lately, she's been unable to find the clothing she needs, so I have amended the routine. She now states what she needs to wear, and I get it for her.

A second, familiar task is setting the table. We discuss the meal we're going to have and decide which plates, bowls, utensils, and napkins are needed. I take out those items as she lists them, and she places them in the correct order on the place mats. If something is missing, she tries, with cues from me, to figure out what it is.

Sequence puzzles offer another option for this type of skill. Cut from a magazine three to four pictures of an event (for example, pictures of an outside party, someone eating food, and someone washing dishes). Mix up the order of the pictures, then ask your parent to place them in order from left to right. Ask him or her to discuss what is going on in the pictures. Cues you can offer may include "Which comes first?" or "What do you think happens next?"

It's important to remember that if sequencing is too frustrating, change what you're doing by reducing the number of steps needed to accomplish it or eliminate it altogether.

Assess This Activity

Date: _____

Name of activity:

_____

Setup location (inside, outside, at a table, in which room):

_____

Setup requirements (where you sat, where your parent sat, type of chairs used, table covering, lighting, any necessary equipment used):

_____

_____

_____

Time of day the activity was done (morning, afternoon, before or after a meal):

_____

Length of time spent at the activity:

_____

Was the activity successful? Did your parent like doing it? Did you?

_____

_____

Did you have to tweak the activity to make it work better for you or your parent? If so, describe how:

_____

_____

Did you teach another person how to do this activity, ensuring you weren't the only one to do it? If so, who?

_____

Would you do this activity again? Yes or no? Why or why not

_____

_____

_____

Shape Sorting

An abundance of shape-sorting toys exist in the marketplace, which you can use with your parent. From flat-surfaced chunky puzzles to large plastic or wooden boxes with cutout shapes on their sides, there are so many to choose from.

Many shape sorters are made of plastic in vibrant colors; some are made from bare wood. With some toys the individual pieces are larger and thicker, making them easier to handle and more visible—I like these best. Some puzzle-shape sorters now come with knobs that are great for those whose hands are afflicted with arthritis.

I have also found that many of these toys vary the quantity of shapes available for sorting. Too many options can cause confusion. I like the toy that includes the basic shapes, those that to your parent are most familiar from childhood. The shapes should include at least the following: a square, a triangle, a circle, a star, a rectangle, an oval, and possibly a pentagon. Your parent's level of cognition will dictate which specific type of shape-sorting toy works best.

Setup for this activity should be at a well-lit table where your parent is comfortably seated. Be sure to cover the surface with a contrasting colored cloth, so when the pieces are poured out, they are easily visible. You can ask your parent to name all the shapes, or if his or her word-finding skills are affected, you can name the shapes for him or her. Ask your parent for a specific shape and have him or her put it into the correct space and continue to completion.

I was doing this shape-sorter activity with my mother when she got to the star piece. She pointed out another star from a coloring page we had done earlier. I then went to find a star pin she often wears. Our discussion turned to stars and the skies at night. It was great.

Assess This Activity

Date: _____

Name of activity:

_____

Setup location (inside, outside, at a table, in which room):

_____

Setup requirements (where you sat, where your parent sat, type of chairs used, table covering, lighting, any necessary equipment used):

_____

_____

_____

Time of day the activity was done (morning, afternoon, before or after a meal):

_____

Length of time spent at the activity:

_____

Was the activity successful? Did your parent like doing it? Did you?

_____

_____

Did you have to tweak the activity to make it work better for you or your parent? If so, describe how:

_____

_____

Did you teach another person how to do this activity, ensuring you weren't the only one to do it? If so, who?

_____

Would you do this activity again? Yes or no? Why or why not

_____

_____

_____

Sing-Along

Years ago there was a TV program called *Sing Along with Mitch*. The country loved Mitch Miller, and I bet your parent did too. The words of his many songs scrolled across the bottom of the screen to encourage audience participation. It was fun, and everyone joined in.

You don't have to provide the words across your living room wall, but singing along with a song is a great activity to do with someone who has dementia. Choose songs that were popular during the years when your parent was younger. You can find many lyrics on the Internet, which can then be printed out in large bold fonts that are easily read. There are also sing-along songbooks that may be found in your library or local music shop. I have also seen Mitch Miller CDs in our local Walmart, Sears, and Best Buy stores.

Consider children's songs as well. They will be familiar to your parent from the time you were small. "The Alphabet Song" is one that might be easily recalled as well as possibly "The Wheels on the Bus" or even "Mary Had a Little Lamb." The grandchildren can certainly participate along with your parent while doing this activity.

For consistency your sing-along should take place at the same time of day and in the same location. Sit next to your parent and, while listening to the appropriate CD, hold a shared lyric sheet of that music selection and start singing. Sing loudly and enjoy yourselves.

Singing encourages breath control. In addition to being fun, it offers a congenial atmosphere. Singing old songs stimulates memory. It encourages conversation. Try it; you'll like it.

Assess This Activity

Date: _____

Name of activity:

_____

Setup location (inside, outside, at a table, in which room):

_____

Setup requirements (where you sat, where your parent sat, type of chairs used, table covering, lighting, any necessary equipment used):

_____

_____

_____

Time of day the activity was done (morning, afternoon, before or after a meal):

_____

Length of time spent at the activity:

_____

Was the activity successful? Did your parent like doing it? Did you?

_____

_____

Did you have to tweak the activity to make it work better for you or your parent? If so, describe how:

_____

_____

Did you teach another person how to do this activity, ensuring you weren't the only one to do it? If so, who?

_____

Would you do this activity again? Yes or no? Why or why not

_____

_____

_____

STEPPING ON STONES

*A*s dementia progresses, individuals display less attention to their surroundings. Their world view gets smaller and becomes even more limited. Increasingly they pay attention only to themselves, and their physical senses remain the driving force for any actions. Are they hungry? Are they too hot? Are they tired? The emphasis is on their own bodies and anything unconnected to them is ignored.

Stepping on Stones is one game that helps to refocus attention away from themselves and outward toward their immediate environment.

My "stones" are made from flat pieces of nonskid material. Some are made from the rubberized mesh carpet backing found in hardware stores, such as K-Mart or Home Depot. I have also made them from mesh place mats and have used the rubberized disks used for jar openers. They are made of multiple colors and shapes. My criteria are that they must be a minimum of six to eight inches wide in a color that differs from the floor beneath them so they are easily seen. They must be made from a nonskid material to prevent falling.

I spread my "stones" across our hard-surfaced floor. Putting them on carpeting is a fall risk since they don't lie flat. The object of the game is to step from one stone to another. At this time my mother is able to follow simple two-step directions. For example, "Find the yellow circle and go stand on it." When her memory was better I could offer more complex instructions. An example of this is "Find the yellow circle, stand on it, and then go to the red square."

The game lasts until fatigue sets in, usually after about fifteen minutes. When we stop, it becomes her turn to direct me in picking up the "stones" so we can put them away. She has to look around the room and select which ones I should retrieve. With cues she must also check to see that all have been collected.

Assess This Activity

Name of activity:

_____

Setup location (inside, outside, at a table, in which room):

_____

Setup requirements (where you sat, where your parent sat, type of chairs used, table covering, lighting, any necessary equipment used):

_____

_____

_____

Time of day the activity was done (morning, afternoon, before or after a meal):

_____

Length of time spent at the activity:

_____

Was the activity successful? Did your parent like doing it? Did you?

_____

_____

Did you have to tweak the activity to make it work better for you or your parent? If so, describe how:

_____

_____

Did you teach another person how to do this activity, ensuring you weren't the only one to do it? If so, who?

_____

Would you do this activity again? Yes or no? Why or why not

_____

_____

_____

STICKERS

Stickers are available everywhere. From the supermarket checkout line with the bright-orange "Paid" stickers to craft shops, such as Michael's, they are available in multitudes of colors, shapes, and textures. I have also been able to find plastic gemstone stickers with a peel off backing.

When I was young, we were thrilled with Colorforms, a malleable material that could adhere to smooth surfaces and then be removed and placed somewhere else. These can still be found in some toy stores. Today, with the onset of scrap booking, stickers are now available in designs that depict any story line, be it animals found on a farm to designer wedding glassware and dresses. There's even a line of puffy googly-eyed stickers for your Halloween pumpkins.

I've found that stickers are presented for sale in three ways. The first is when they are die-cut from a sheet of paper and left in place. This method necessitates finding the edge of the sticker and then being able to fold it back from the paper for removal. This step can be difficult for someone with decreased vision or fine hand-control problems that may be due to arthritis or tremors. When I purchase this type of sticker, it means I'm the remover of the stickers and that I have to hand them to my mother.

The second way stickers are sold is when they have been die-cut and then repositioned on a different sheet of paper. The area around this type of sticker is flat, which makes them easier to see and remove. However, these are usually the more ornate ones and thus are often more expensive.

The third kind of presentation I have found is individually cutout foam stickers sold by the container. These are the most economical. I have seen them in Michael's craft shops. While they are easy to hold, they still require you or the caretaker to peel off the backing to enable you to use them.

The stickers I choose to use with my mother take her visual limitations into account. I look for stickers that are large, brightly colored, and textured. When possible, I prefer her to be able to remove the sticker backing. The exercise then becomes more her task than mine.

We have placed stickers on anything and everything! We've made stationery, with them as the decoration. We have adorned jewelry boxes. We have placed them on door hangers. We have covered picture frames with them. We have placed them on foam hat visors. And since they can be bought by theme, I have used them to initiate story lines.

Assess This Activity

Date: _____

Name of activity:

_____

Setup location (inside, outside, at a table, in which room):

_____

Setup requirements (where you sat, where your parent sat, type of chairs used, table covering, lighting, any necessary equipment used):

_____

_____

_____

Time of day the activity was done (morning, afternoon, before or after a meal):

_____

Length of time spent at the activity:

_____

Was the activity successful? Did your parent like doing it? Did you?

_____

_____

Did you have to tweak the activity to make it work better for you or your parent? If so, describe how:

_____

_____

Did you teach another person how to do this activity, ensuring you weren't the only one to do it? If so, who?

_____

Would you do this activity again? Yes or no? Why or why not

_____

_____

_____

STORYTELLING

I went to my mother's house with the intention of getting her to initiate the telling of a story. This isn't easy to do since people suffering with dementia frequently require an outside stimulus to begin any activity.

I thought I would start by telling her a story, a familiar one to her from the past, and decided to use a fairy tale. I chose the "Three Bears" and proceeded as far as "Once upon a time there were three bears: the papa bear, the mama bear and" when she jumped in with "the baby bear." I continued to relate the rest of the story, and my mother was able to fill in each story line as the tale progressed. While this activity was good and filled time in a purposeful way, her response wasn't my intention. I wanted her to initiate the story, not just fill in the blanks.

I said to my mother, "I've told you a story. Now you tell me one." Her immediate reply was no. I was stumped. The problem was that I had failed to provide the necessary stimulus to get her started. I rephrased my request as "It's your turn to tell me a story." I then said, "Once upon a time," and she began.

Her story was "Once upon a time there was a young girl who worked very hard to earn her money. She worked in a department store and sold slips." Since my mother had a very good friend who had manufactured lingerie, the story was put on hold while we spoke about her friend. Also, as a young woman, my mother had worked in a department store. We discussed this experience as well. When we exhausted those topics, I went back and reviewed her earlier story. She was able to continue and added a few more sentences until she determined she was done.

Assess This Activity

Date: _____

Name of activity:

_____

Setup location (inside, outside, at a table, in which room):

_____

Setup requirements (where you sat, where your parent sat, type of chairs used, table covering, lighting, any necessary equipment used):

_____

_____

_____

Time of day the activity was done (morning, afternoon, before or after a meal):

_____

Length of time spent at the activity:

_____

Was the activity successful? Did your parent like doing it? Did you?

_____

_____

Did you have to tweak the activity to make it work better for you or your parent? If so, describe how:

_____

_____

Did you teach another person how to do this activity, ensuring you weren't the only one to do it? If so, who?

_____

Would you do this activity again? Yes or no? Why or why not

_____

_____

_____

TIC TAC TOE

ic Tac Toe is one of those old-fashioned games that probably originated before your parent was born. It is surely in his or her long-term memory bank and something he or she would willingly like to play. In addition, it is a wonderful game for your parent when you want him or her to interact with the grandchildren. Keep score to see who wins. Don't be surprised if the winner turns out to be your parent!

I like this game; we can play anywhere. Setup is simple, and cost is negligible. Because of my mother's visual limitations, I prefer to use bright, white paper for the background and to write with dark markers: black for one side and red for the other. I make sure to draw a large grid so it is clearly visible. For those with arthritic hands, I have found that large markers are easiest to hold. I have also played this game using the red or black disks from her checkers game. These work well for those people who lack the hand coordination necessary to write yet still enjoy and benefit from playing.

Tic Tac Toe is a game that encourages decision-making skills. My mother has to choose whether she is X or O as well as which color marker she will use. I also let her decide which one of us will go first. She has to determine where she will place her mark. She has to notice when either of us has won. Should we play again, she has to remember who the previous winner was. Only then can she determine who gets to start next.

Assess This Activity

Name of activity:

_____

Setup location (inside, outside, at a table, in which room):

_____

Setup requirements (where you sat, where your parent sat, type of chairs used, table covering, lighting, any necessary equipment used):

_____

_____

_____

Time of day the activity was done (morning, afternoon, before or after a meal):

_____

Length of time spent at the activity:

_____

Was the activity successful? Did your parent like doing it? Did you?

_____

_____

Did you have to tweak the activity to make it work better for you or your parent? If so, describe how:

_____

_____

Did you teach another person how to do this activity, ensuring you weren't the only one to do it? If so, who?

_____

Would you do this activity again? Yes or no? Why or why not

_____

_____

_____

WALKING

$\mathcal{J}$t sounds simple, but just going for a walk can be easily overlooked. It remains a wonderful exercise for all ages and all abilities. Whether to walk independently, with the use of a cane, with a walker, or even with a wheelchair, it is so good to be mobile. Often older people are more sensitive to the cold, so if you take a walk outside, ensure that they're dressed appropriately and wear well-fitting shoes. Then extend your arm, point the way, and get moving.

If your walk will be indoors, the hallway in your building may be considered one place to go. It provides a sheltered, level surface, and you can easily return home if necessary. Consider placing a chair in the hallway to use as a rest stop in case it is needed. Endurance and stamina can be improved when a routine exercise program is included in your day.

Walking on uneven surfaces, such as an outside sidewalk, offers more physical challenges since better balance and longer endurance are required. You can progress from one area to the next depending on ability. You can also increase the length of the walk as your goal. Just remember that after you get to your destination, you have to be able to get back.

A location where I often go with my mother is the mall. The walking surface is level, and there are plenty of seating areas available in case of fatigue. The varied stores offer visual interest, and we can easily set our direction. There is also an indoor children's gym area she likes to visit. She gets great pleasure from watching them play.

There was a period of time this past winter when my mother required the use of a wheelchair. Her endurance level became poor, but we still wanted her to get some exercise. She was able to push the wheelchair until she tired, and then she sat in it while we pushed her throughout the mall. As her stamina improved, the wheelchair was returned to the car trunk and now to the hall closet. It is ready to be used again when necessary.

Something to consider when walking is whether to carry any items. Women love their handbags, but they are often heavy and can cause walking imbalances. Consider instead a shoulder bag worn across the chest, a fanny pack that buckles around the waist, or even an apron with a large pocket where items can be held. It might be just what your parent needs to feel most stable.

Walking provides a change from the routine of being inside all day. It offers openings for conversation. You can discuss the weather, describe if it's cloudy, sunny, cold, or hot. Discuss the seasons; discuss what type of clothing is required for each season. Have your parent list what he or she is wearing and then try to figure out what the season happens to be. Have him or her name the months of each season or even try to name a holiday that falls into each time frame. Anything is open for discussion, from cars on the road to a car he or she might have owned in the past. It's not a quiz; just have fun.

Assess This Activity

Date: _____

Name of activity:

_____

Setup location (inside, outside, at a table, in which room):

_____

Setup requirements (where you sat, where your parent sat, type of chairs used, table covering, lighting, any necessary equipment used):

_____

_____

_____

Time of day the activity was done (morning, afternoon, before or after a meal):

_____

Length of time spent at the activity:

_____

Was the activity successful? Did your parent like doing it? Did you?

_____

_____

Did you have to tweak the activity to make it work better for you or your parent? If so, describe how:

_____

_____

Did you teach another person how to do this activity, ensuring you weren't the only one to do it? If so, who?

_____

Would you do this activity again? Yes or no? Why or why not

_____

_____

_____

WATCHING TELEVISION

*T*elevision offers an abundance of stimulation for an individual with dementia. Rapidly changing visual images as well as vivid colors can attract and hold attention. Programs you might consider too juvenile are often appropriate for a parent with dementia.

During daytime television the repetitive sing-song nature of *Sesame Street, Nickelodeon,* or even *Barney* can provide reminders of basic relationships, the weather, and the alphabet. These shows are nonthreatening and offer familiarity as the structure of the program remains constant. Each segment is of short duration and frequently uses songs to reinforce the concepts being taught. The characters are usually depicted in bright colors and are easily recognized. This type of programming is directed toward the viewer and encourages interaction. An evening news broadcast that offers a listing of events with an anchor sitting behind a news desk doesn't function in this same manner.

With the advent of cable television, many more channels are now available. Finding an appropriate show all day, every day, is easy. Reality TV has now become the norm, and with it dancing and singing shows have become prevalent. This type of show is wonderful too for the person with dementia to watch. Each song and/or dance segment is of limited duration and presented along with glitzy costuming and background designs. It is perfect for someone with shortened attention span.

Though stimulation from television can be beneficial, it can also be a distraction when your parent is trying to concentrate on something else. Remember to turn off the television when your parent is trying to attend to another activity.

Assess This Activity

Date: _____

Name of activity:

_____

Setup location (inside, outside, at a table, in which room):

_____

Setup requirements (where you sat, where your parent sat, type of chairs used, table covering, lighting, any necessary equipment used):

_____

_____

_____

Time of day the activity was done (morning, afternoon, before or after a meal):

_____

Length of time spent at the activity:

_____

Was the activity successful? Did your parent like doing it? Did you?

_____

_____

Did you have to tweak the activity to make it work better for you or your parent? If so, describe how:

_____

_____

Did you teach another person how to do this activity, ensuring you weren't the only one to do it? If so, who?

_____

Would you do this activity again? Yes or no? Why or why not

_____

_____

_____

WINDING YARN

I am a crocheter, and my mother had always loved to do needlepoint. Needless to say, we have a huge amount of leftover yarn in both of our homes. The colors don't match. The type of yarn varies, but that doesn't matter. Simply take one end and wind the yarn into a ball. When you finish with one color, just tie on the next. The motion is repetitive and easy to do. Familiarity breeds comfort.

While we wrap, I ask my mother the color of the yarn she's using. If she has difficulty coming up with the name, I offer a clue as to what it might be. An example of this is when she might be winding with red yarn. I ask her, "What is your favorite lipstick color?" or "What colors are cherries?" This is often the trigger she needs to come up with the answer. We continue on until we get to another color, and then we do it again.

There is a craft project I have done with my children called "A God's Eye." This is a good project for my mother to do with them. To make it, you will need two sticks (we have used chopsticks, pencils, and even branches from the backyard), yarn, and a pair of scissors.

Lay the sticks across each other to form a plus sign. Secure the sticks in this position by tying them with your chosen yarn. Once they are tightly secured, start by placing a loop of yarn around the top stick. Do this one time. Then, moving counterclockwise, bring the yarn to the next stick and wrap a loop around that. Continue wrapping until you get back to the first loop. Repeat this process, pressing the loops toward the center for the best look until you get to your desired size or decide to change the yarn color. Tie on another color and keep going. If you decide to stop, simply knot the yarn at that point and use the scissors to trim the edge.

Assess This Activity

Date: _____

Name of activity:

_____

Setup location (inside, outside, at a table, in which room):

_____

Setup requirements (where you sat, where your parent sat, type of chairs used, table covering, lighting, any necessary equipment used):

_____

_____

_____

Time of day the activity was done (morning, afternoon, before or after a meal):

_____

Length of time spent at the activity:

_____

Was the activity successful? Did your parent like doing it? Did you?

_____

_____

Did you have to tweak the activity to make it work better for you or your parent? If so, describe how:

_____

_____

Did you teach another person how to do this activity, ensuring you weren't the only one to do it? If so, who?

_____

Would you do this activity again? Yes or no? Why or why not

_____

_____

_____

WORD FIND

On a daily basis our local newspaper offers the "Word Find" game. A specific word is presented along with its definition. The task is to find a set number of words created of four or more letters within a defined time limit. My mother has always loved this game. I have tweaked it a bit to work within her limitations, and she still enjoys playing this game.

You can choose the word, or your parent can select a word that is familiar to him or her. Since my mother's name is composed of nine letters, I have at times chosen that as our word. She then tries to make as many words as she can using the letters within her name. It doesn't matter how many letters are in her words—two, three, or more. As she says them, I write them down. No duplicates are allowed. When she repeats a word, we review our list to see if it already appears. If so, I don't write it down. Invariably she's able to come up with another word, and we continue on.

Assess This Activity

Date: _____

Name of activity:

_____

Setup location (inside, outside, at a table, in which room):

_____

Setup requirements (where you sat, where your parent sat, type of chairs used, table covering, lighting, any necessary equipment used):

_____

_____

_____

Time of day the activity was done (morning, afternoon, before or after a meal):

_____

Length of time spent at the activity:

_____

Was the activity successful? Did your parent like doing it? Did you?

_____

_____

Did you have to tweak the activity to make it work better for you or your parent? If so, describe how:

_____

_____

Did you teach another person how to do this activity, ensuring you weren't the only one to do it? If so, who?

_____

Would you do this activity again? Yes or no? Why or why not

_____

_____

_____

WRITING AND DRAWING

My mother still has the ability to write. She does, however, have some difficulty with vision. So if we want to practice writing or drawing, I use a Sharpie or a black marker in place of a regular pen. These are large enough to be easily held, and the lines they make are thick and easily seen. The paper color we use is either white or ivory, which offers good visual contrast.

I seat myself within my mother's visual range to be certain she can see what I'm writing. I prefer to sit to her left—in this instance since this is a left-to-right skill. If your parent is unable to see to that side, you can still stay there (reinforcing him or her to look to that side) but place your sample directly in front of your parent and have him or her copy it on a second paper placed to its right.

I initiate the specific drawing task I want my mother to do. I make sure that my instructions are clearly stated and understood before beginning.

My mother and I have drawn shapes. We have drawn circles and turned them into clocks. We follow with a discussion of time and of whether she is hungry or whether it's before or after lunch. We have also drawn circles and turned them into faces, making sure all parts are included—eyes, eyebrows, nose, mouth, ears, and hair. Since she's always wearing earrings, I make sure those are added as well. We have drawn stick figures, taking care to ensure all arms and legs are properly placed.

Initially the drawings were more complicated—a stick figure on a sunny day that included the sun, trees, and flowers. Now we do the body parts. As with other activities, if this is too difficult or causes frustration, stop, change the task, and reassess what you're doing. This is supposed to be fun, not art class. You want your parent to succeed, and you want to have a good time while being together.

We have written the letters of the alphabet. I always emphasize the letters of her name. She can copy me as I write, and with cues she can write her name on her own.

Lately my mother's vision has further decreased, and I've needed her to sign some forms. I've taken a black piece of paper and cut from it a rectangular shape, approximately one inch by three inches. I use this template as a frame. I place it over the paper where she needs to sign her name; it defines the area where she must write. It works quite well.

Assess This Activity

Date: _____

Name of activity:

_____

Setup location (inside, outside, at a table, in which room):

_____

Setup requirements (where you sat, where your parent sat, type of chairs used, table covering, lighting, any necessary equipment used):

_____

_____

_____

Time of day the activity was done (morning, afternoon, before or after a meal):

_____

Length of time spent at the activity:

_____

Was the activity successful? Did your parent like doing it? Did you?

_____

_____

Did you have to tweak the activity to make it work better for you or your parent? If so, describe how:

_____

_____

Did you teach another person how to do this activity, ensuring you weren't the only one to do it? If so, who?

_____

Would you do this activity again? Yes or no? Why or why not

_____

_____

_____

RESOURCES

DEFINITIONS

Activities of Daily Living (ADL)—Everyday self-care activities individuals perform. The six basic areas include eating, bathing, dressing, toileting, transferring or walking, and continence.

Alzheimer's Dementia (AD)—This is the most common form of dementia. It usually occurs in old age. It's marked by a decline in cognitive functions, such as remembering, reasoning, and planning.

Attention Span—The length of time a person can concentrate on a subject or idea and remain interested.

Burnout or Caregiver Burnout—Exhaustion of physical or emotional strength or motivation usually as a result of prolonged stress or frustration.

Cognition—The mental process of knowing; it includes awareness, perception, reasoning, and judgment.

Dementia—The loss of mental ability that is severe enough to interfere with normal activities of daily living.

It is not present since birth, lasts longer than six months, and isn't associated with a loss or change in consciousness. Other symptoms include decreased judgment, language, and memory.

Instrumental Activities of Daily Living (IADL)— Activities not necessary for basic functioning but needed for an individual to live independently within a community. They include shopping, housework, accounting, food preparation or medications, telephone, or transportation.

Memory—The mental process of retaining and recalling past experiences over time.

Perception—The ability to interpret sensations that allow us to make sense of the world around us.

Peripheral Vision—The part of vision that occurs outside of the very center of one's gaze; side vision.

Sensation—Awareness of our environment through the sense of touch, taste, sight, sound, and smell.

Sequencing—The ability to place items in order.

Sundowning—An increase in agitation and delusional behavior with the onset of dusk. Seen in individuals with cognitive loss and most frequently in those with Alzheimer's dementia.

Tactile—Of or related to the sensation of touch.

Tactile Discrimination—The ability to differentiate between objects using just the sense of touch.

Visual Field—The entire area that can be seen when the eye is directed forward.

ACTIVITY RESOURCES

Amazing Savings
http://www.amazingsavings.com

Amazon
http://www.amazon.com

eBay
http://www.ebay.com

Fisher-Price Toys
http://www.fisher-price.com

Guidecraft Toys
http://www.fatbraintoys.com

Melissa & Doug Toys
http://www.melissaanddoug.com

Michaels Craft Stores
http://www.michaels.com

National Mah Jongg League
http://www.nationalmahjonggleague.org

ALZHEIMER'S RESOURCES

Albert Einstein College of Medicine
Einstein Aging Study
1300 Morris Peck Ave.
Bronx, NY 10461
Telephone: 718-430-2000
information@einstein.yu.edu

Alzheimer's Association National Office
25 N. Michigan Ave., 17th Floor
Chicago, IL 60601
Help Line: 1-800-272-3900
http://www.alz.org

Alzheimer's Disease Education and Referral Center (ADEAR)
PO Box 8250
Silver Spring, MD 20907
Telephone: 1-800-438-4380
http://www.nia.nih.gov/alzheimers

Alzheimer's Disease Research Foundation
1236 Ginger Crescent
Virginia Beach, VA 23453
Telephone: 1-877-427-0220
http://www.alzheimers-research.org

Alzheimer's Foundation of America (AFA)
322 8th Ave., 7th Floor
New York, NY 10001
Telephone: 1-866-232-8484
http://www.alzfdn.org
http://www.alzquilt.org

Arts & Minds
Connect2culture
PO Box 250073
Columbia University Station
New York, NY 10025
Telephone: 646-873-0712
http://www.artsandminds.org

Bright Focus Foundation
(Formerly American Health Assistance Foundation)
22512 Gateway Center Dr.
Clarksburg, MD 20871
Telephone: 1-800-437-2423
http://www.brightfocus.org

Family Caregiver Alliance
785 Market St., Ste. 750
San Francisco, CA 94103
Telephone: 1-800-445-8106
http://www.caregiving.org

Keep Memory Alive
Cleveland Clinic Lou Ruvo Center for Brain Health
888 W. Bonneville Ave.
Las Vegas, NV 89106
Telephone for Support Groups: 702-331-7042
louruvosocialserv@ccf.org

Medicare Hotline
Telephone: 1-800-633-4227
http://www.medicare.gov

Music & Memory
160 First St.
PO Box 590
Mineola, NY 11501
info@musicandmemory.org

National Adult Day Services Association (NADSA)
2519 Connecticut Ave., NW
Washington, DC 20008
Telephone: 1-800-558-5301
http://www.nadsa.org

National Eldercare Locator
Telephone: 1-800-677-1116
http://www.n4a.org/programs/eldercare-locator

National Family Caregivers Association (NFCA)
10400 Connecticut Ave., Ste. 500
Kensington, MD 20895-3944
Telephone: 1-800-896-3650
http://www.thefamilycaregiver.org

National Hospice and Palliative Care Organization (NHPCO)
1700 Diagonal Rd., Ste. 625
Alexandria, VA 22314
Telephone: 703-837-1500
http://www.nhpco.org

National Institute on Aging
Bldg. 31, Rm. 5C27
31 Center Dr., MSC 2292
Bethesda, MD 20892
Telephone: 301-496-1752
http://www.nia.nih.gov

Penn State Hershey Medical Center
Memory & Cognitive Disorders Clinic
500 University Dr.
Hershey, PA 17003
Telephone: 1-800-243-1455
http://www.pennstatehershey.org

Social Security Administration
Telephone: 1-800-772-1213
http://www.ssa.gov

Validation Training Institute, Inc.
21987 Byron Rd.
Cleveland, OH 44122
Telephone: 216-921-6606

PREVENTING CAREGIVER BURNOUT

When you are a caregiver, you need to acknowledge that there might come a time when your parent's needs are more than you can handle. The continuing needs of a parent with Alzheimer's dementia might be greater than your physical, emotional, and financial capabilities. Studies have shown that caretakers of Alzheimer's patients may have a decreased life expectancy. You need to step back and assess how you're handling yourself and your parent.

Some specific questions to ask yourself include the following:

- Are you torn between your role as caregiver and your roles as a spouse, parent, child, or friend?
- Do you feel you are directing all your energy toward taking care of someone else?
- Do you feel guilty for being frustrated, angry, and stressed?
- Do you wonder where the "me" time went?

Some symptoms of caregiver burnout include the following:

- Withdrawal from friends and family;
- Loss of interest in activities you previously enjoyed;
- Feelings of irritableness and helplessness;
- Changes in appetite or weight or both;
- Changes in sleep patterns;
- More frequent sickness;
- Desire to hurt yourself or the person you're caring for;
- Emotional and physical exhaustion; and
- Increased use of alcohol or sleep aids or both.

Some tools to prevent caregiver burnout include the following:

- Join a caregiver support group.
- Set reasonable limits.
- Take care of your own health.
- Make time for outside activities you enjoy.
- Reach out for help.

Outside services might be beneficial to alleviate your stress. Contacts to consider include home health services, adult daycare, nursing homes, assisted-living facilities, private-care aides, your local Agency on Aging, AARP, and national organizations specific to Alzheimer's disease. Check in your local yellow pages under "Senior Services".

Home and Personal Safety Assessment

Does my parent have problems with balance? If so, I should consider
- their need for a cane or walker;
- their need to walk with help; and
- their need to have handrails installed on their stairs.

Does my parent rush to the bathroom? If so, I should consider
- their need to wear a pad or diaper;
- their need to toilet on a schedule; and
- their need for a bedside commode or urinal.

Could my parent's medications cause a fall? If so, I should consider
- their medication schedule;
- whether they are taking diuretics, laxatives, pain medicines, sleeping pills, blood pressure or anxiety medications which can contribute to falls;
- their need to stand and change positions slowly;

- their need to use the same pharmacy;
- their medication's side effects, especially if they are taking more than four pills a day;
- their need for a doctor visit to review continuing or revising their medications and, reinforcing precautions and food interactions; their need to know what their pills are for.

Is my parent's home safe? If not, I should consider
- their need to have clear pathways;
- their need to have pets contained;
- their need to have handrails installed on the stairs;
- their need to have a handrail installed in the bathtub;
- their need to have arm rails installed on the toilet;
- their need to use a shower seat or tub bench;
- their need for nonskid strips in the tub;
- their need to remove loose rugs; and
- their need to remove dangerous cords.

Does my parent wander? If so, I should consider
- the need to keep personal identification inside his or her shoe or on his or her cell phone;
- the need to notify the local police to be aware of him or her; and
- the need for secure front-door locks which are difficult to open.

What else can my parent do to be safer?
- wear eyeglasses when walking, if needed;

- have help with bathing, if needed;
- have a medical alert device and/or cordless phone that is preprogrammed with emergency contact numbers, and keep it on him or her;
- visit his or her doctor at least once a year;
- wear flat, proper fitting rubber-soled shoes or slippers;
- rearrange items on shelves to prevent stretching for objects;
- use a night-light;
- use his or her cane or walker appropriately;
- keep a list next to his or her phone and in his or her wallet that provides names and phone numbers of doctors, names of medications with dosages and, emergency contacts;
- write down his or her address and keep it next to his or her phone so in an emergency he or she knows where he or she is; and
- review and write down plans for future living arrangements and apprise family and legal advisers of their location.

Room-by-Room Home Safety Suggestions

Bathroom

Install grab railings by the tub, shower, and toilet. Use adhesive nonskid strips in the tub and shower. Eliminate scatter rugs and replace with nonskid carpeting. Use a padded shower seat and handheld shower head to make bathing safer and more convenient. Keep a cell phone or baby monitor nearby when taking a shower.

Bedroom

Keep nighttime temperature above sixty-five degrees. Place telephones and light switches within reach of the bed. Obtain and keep a medical alert device near your bed. Before getting up from bed, sit on its side for a few minutes before standing. This step helps to avoid dizziness.

Entry/Exits

Place childproof or wander-proof locks on all doors.

Kitchen

Keep items used every day within close range to avoid excessive reaching, bending, and stooping. Keep lighter objects on higher shelves. Eliminate scatter rugs and replace with nonskid carpeting. Use a rolling tea cart to carry items from the stove or oven to the table. Place a written list of medications with a dosage schedule inside a marked plastic container in the refrigerator. Place a decal on the refrigerator door, showing where this container may be found.

Lighting

Good lighting is important in every room of the house. Make sure the brightness is adequate to see clearly. Install light switches at the entrance and exit to every room. Ensure that the entrance to your house has adequate lighting as well. Put outside lighting on a timer.

Living Room

Keep cords and telephone wires out of the way. Cover slippery surfaces with nonskid carpeting. Remove any scatter rugs. Make sure there is a color contrast between the furniture and the walls. Place a colored afghan over the back of the sofa to help define its location and prevent bumping into walls, which might lead to falls and bruising.

Stairs

Install railings on both sides of the stairs. Mark the first and last steps with brightly colored tape. Make sure there are light switches at both the top and the bottom of the stairs. On outside stairs apply gritty, weatherproof paint on the steps.

Telephones

Install extensions and cordless phones in as many rooms as possible. Adjust the volume on the speaker so you can hear easily. Keep emergency contact numbers and your home address next to your phones.

ABOUT THE AUTHOR

*J*udith A. Levy, EdM, OTR, graduated from Sargent College of Allied Health Professions, Boston University, where she received her bachelor of science degree in occupational therapy. She is also a graduate of Rutgers University with a master's degree in Allied Health Education. She has worked for more than forty years as an occupational therapist.

Her primary focus has been in the area of adult rehabilitation. She has established occupational therapy departments in community hospitals and has worked in acute-care hospitals, assisted-living centers, long-term care facilities, and home care settings. She has also spent time working with developmentally delayed children in institutions, school settings, summer camps, and home-based environments.

Mrs. Levy has been an instructor teaching occupational therapy skills to home health aides as part of their certification process and has been a guest lecturer for a local college's occupational therapy program.

She can be contacted at: dementiaactivities@gmail.com.

CPSIA information can be obtained
at www.ICGtesting.com
Printed in the USA
BVHW01s1825170118
505573BV00003B/26/P

9 781491 016442